PRIMARY CARE DEVELOPMENT

Managing the Practice

whose business?

June Huntington
Independent Consultant and Part-time Fellow
King's Fund College, London

Foreword by **Ken Jarrold**
Director of Human Resources
NHS Executive Headquarters, Leeds

Series Editors **Pat Gordon** and **Diane Plamping**

Published in association with King's Fund, London

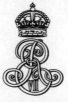

Radcliffe Medical Press
Oxford and New York

Radcliffe Medical Press Ltd
18 Marcham Road, Abingdon, Oxon OX14 1AA, UK

Radcliffe Medical Press, Inc.
141 Fifth Avenue, New York, NY 10010, USA

British Library Cataloguing in Publication Data

A Catalogue record for this book is available from the British Library.

ISBN 185775 053 5

Library of Congress Cataloging-in-Publication Data is available.

Typeset by AMA Graphics Ltd, Preston
Printed in Great Britain by BPC Wheatons Ltd, Exeter

Contents

Series introduction

Primary care development is arguably the most important topic for the NHS to get to grips with in the rapidly changing environment of the 1990s. This new series of books about primary care development is intended to be topical, useful and, before very long, out-of-date. It is based on the current work of the King's Fund Primary Care Group and the ideas, experience and inspiration of a number of people who have worked with us and shared their enthusiasms.

Primary care is often used to mean general practice. Here it is used in the broader sense to include the network of community-based health services which in the UK allow us to manage 90% of care outside hospitals; to manage earlier, safer discharge from hospitals, and to maintain people at home who do not want to be institutionalized.

From a position of relative neglect and invisibility, primary care has shot to the top of the NHS policy agenda. This has much to do with the NHS reforms and the drive to control public spending. Like all industrialized nations faced with ever-increasing costs in health care, we are experimenting with reorganization. Since hospitals use most NHS resources, this is where most attention was directed and primary care became the focus only as a potentially cheaper option. But the drive for efficiency and value for money coincides with other powerful influences which challenge us to examine alternatives to traditional ways of delivering services. If effective primary care really is the key to successful health services in the future, then recognizing its distinctive characteristics, and what we value about it as well as what we want to change becomes critical. In other words, primary care has development needs in its own right quite apart from the current emphasis on the shift from secondary to primary care – the so-called substitution agenda.

This new series is about ideas and services which are being developed and tested around the country. It is about work-in-progress in a period of extraordinary change. *Managing the Practice: whose business?* is the second title in the series. It is about the development of general practices as primary care organizations. Its starting point is that a health service which is primary care led will require effectively managed practices. But what does this look like? What does management mean in practice-based primary care? June Huntington's analysis takes us a long way from concerns about 'bureaucracy, control and paperwork' to questions such as why do patients experience some practices as helpful, caring and therapeutic, in the way that a person might be? And why does it matter? We hope the questions and the ideas in this series contribute to the debate about the future shape of the NHS and prove useful to the people now working in the middle of these major changes.

Pat Gordon
King's Fund
London
June 1995

Foreword

June Huntington's study of practice management is valuable for seven reasons. First, because primary care is the bedrock of the NHS. The UK system of general practice has long been established at the centre of the provision of primary care. Following the NHS reforms general practice is now also playing a leading role in the purchasing of hospital and community services.

Second, June's study emphasizes the importance of the management function within general practice. Practices are significant organizations in their own right and good quality practice management is of great importance to the NHS.

Third, the study is based on discussion with GPs and practice managers. It is, therefore, practical and based in reality. This is not a theoretical study. June's book is about, and speaks to, the real world.

Fourth, June highlights the importance of the gender issues in practice management. All those who are committed to good quality management and to the development of people must have a strong commitment to equal opportunities.

Fifth, the study focuses strongly on management development and the learning needs of GPs and practice managers. The emphasis on mentoring is very welcome.

Sixth, the study is based on two Health Commissions in Wessex which are at the leading edge of the development of purchasing. I am proud to have been associated with these Health Commissions in my former role as Chief Executive of the Wessex Regional Health Authority.

Seventh, June guides us through this important subject in the thoughtful and expert manner that has won her widespread respect in the NHS.

Managing the Practice: whose business? is a valuable contribution to our understanding of a vital aspect of the work of the NHS.

Ken Jarrold
Director of Human Resources
NHS Executive Headquarters

June 1995

Acknowledgements

This book is based on a series of workshops attended by over 150 general medical practitioners and their practice managers from two counties of Wessex during the period November 1993 to March 1994.

At the time, Wessex Regional Health Authority had expressed its intention to make primary care the principal focus for health and had encouraged the early development of integrated purchasing through the establishment of health commissions. Two of these, in Dorset and North and Mid Hampshire, together with the NHS Women's Unit recognized that the development of a primary-care-led service would require effectively managed practices.

Consequently, they commissioned a research project which was designed to produce an in-depth picture of the professional and organizational dynamics surrounding the development of management in practice-based primary care. Thanks are due to chief executives Kate Barnard and Ian Carruthers and to Caroline Langridge and Regina Shakespeare for their vision in commissioning the work, and to Annette Clayson and Denis Elkins for their continued interest and support throughout the project.

My personal appreciation goes to those who helped set up and facilitate the workshops which produced so many insights into the current and potential future state of practice management. Fran Ross, then Training Manager of the Hampshire FHSA, and Eleanor Brown, Practice Developments Manager and Consultant in a large fundholding practice in South London co-facilitated the Hampshire workshops, while Howard Nattrass, Dean of the Institute of Health and Community Studies at Bournemouth University and Guy Pettigrew, then Assistant Primary Care Manager at the Dorset health commission, co-facilitated those in Dorset. In post-workshop debriefing sessions, all bore with great patience my protracted attempts to make up for my inability to be in every small group.

The workshops could not have been as productive without the administrative and moral support of Vanessa Casey in Dorset and Sheila Hobden in Hampshire. They approached the administrative complexities of a complex research design with enthusiasm and unflagging interest.

All of those mentioned above would wish to join me in expressing our appreciation of the enthusiastic involvement of the general practitioners and practice managers who took time out from very demanding practice lives to attend two one-day workshops each. The frankness with which they discussed their feelings and perceptions was deeply appreciated. I can only hope that my reporting of them in the aggregate does not unnecessarily violate the feelings and views of any one individual. Similarly, the interpretations placed upon their comments are entirely my responsibility.

Finally, I owe a particular debt of gratitude to my King's Fund colleagues Pat Gordon and Diane Plamping as series editors, and to those at Radcliffe Medical Press whose patience throughout a period of considerable personal stress was deeply appreciated.

Introduction

This book has been written at a time of unprecedented focus on primary health care and on general-practice-based primary health care in particular. The government has espoused its commitment to a primary-care-led NHS and to a 'strategic shift' from secondary to primary care. As those charged with implementing these intentions, some NHS managers, particularly those in the inner city and outer ring areas of the major cities, find the prospect not a little daunting.

General practitioners (GPs), although many deny it, are remarkably free to shape their own organizations. In recent years, however, as government's interest in primary care has intensified, GPs have found that other groups and organizations are beginning to feel that they have or should have a stake in shaping those organizations.

Predominant among these are practice managers. Practice management is one of the fastest growing health care occupations in the UK. Although its members are not employees of the NHS, their salaries are largely financed by it. They are employed by general practitioners and so far most are women who have been appointed from the ranks of practice staff. With the introduction of the 1990 GP Contract and more particularly of fundholding, men are now entering the occupation in greater numbers.

The occupation is typified by a large variety of educational attainment, expertise and former work experience, which adds to the difficulty of developing a focused, assertive occupational association that can identify, represent and promote the corporate interests of such a varied membership. Practice managers also typically occupy a singular role within organizations owned by the GPs who practice medicine within them.

As independent contractors and employers, GPs in their own practices, like Alice in Wonderland, can take the word 'management' and make it mean whatever they choose it to mean. In practice management, as in their clinical work which is shared with other professionals, they are in a position to determine who does what.

Until 1990 their freedom to do this was relatively untrammelled, but as Family Health Service Authorities (FHSAs) were required to extend the range and quality of the Family Practitioner Services, they too began to develop a stake in practice management and its development. In view of the increasing expenditure upon a growing number of practice managers, FHSAs increasingly sought to influence their recruitment, utilization and development.

The new health authorities that will be created in April 1996 with specific government directives to engage in developing, supporting and monitoring practices will have even more reason to stake *their* claim to influence 'the business' (in its broadest definition) of practice management.

The other major stakeholders in this 'business', who are becoming increasingly willing to voice complaint, are patients. Their stake in practice management is not the focus of this book, which is based on material from workshops that did not involve patients and which were focused on changes in practice organization and management *as perceived by GPs and their practice managers.*

GP and practice manager pairs from practices in two health commission areas were recruited to attend two one-day workshops each. From each area, four workshop groups were formed based on practice size, providing a total of two groups of GPs and practice managers from small practices (one to two partners), two groups from practices of three to five partners, two from those of six or more partners and two from fundholding practices. Most of the work was done in three small groups within each workshop, one comprising GPs, the second comprising practice managers, and the third a mix of GPs and practice managers. In all, over 150 GPs and practice managers participated.

The questions addressed were:

- What is the nature of the management function in practice-based primary care?

- How is this currently addressed in your practice? Who does what?

- With what degree of effectiveness?

- What will practice-based primary care look like in five years time?

- In what ways will the management function change?

- What will you need in order to meet this future effectively – capacities, skills, competencies?

- What experiences/events have contributed to your development as a manager? (Participants encouraged to identify life and work experiences not simply formal training/courses.)

- What do you currently feel you need in order to become a more effective manager?

- Develop and work up in small groups a management development activity you feel would address one or more of these needs.

The workshop format was chosen because it brought GPs and practice managers out of their practices for two days and enabled them to discuss the above issues with other GPs and practice managers. It was hoped that the events would not simply provide data for the project but would be experienced as developmental by the participants. Most participants felt they offered a valuable opportunity to develop a better understanding of the NHS changes and of where practice-based primary care, general practice and practice management were headed, and to work through some powerful feelings about these.

Participants were very frank about their feelings about management, their experiences of it and about their need to feel more managerially competent and confident in anticipating the futures they described.

The management function

Introduction

It is often said that general practice is 'demand-led'. Many GPs argue that patients set limits on any attempt to manage general practice more effectively and efficiently. They claim that demand is unpredictable, quoting the emergencies that play havoc with busy surgeries and practice meetings alike. Appointment systems were introduced to give GPs and their organizations more control over the pattern of that demand and their own response to it. In some practices, however, they are increasingly seen as part of the problem rather than its solution. Some practices suffer a high proportion of 'no shows' together with an increasing number of calls out of hours, while others return to open surgeries as a means of mopping up 'excess' demand.

Practices which carry out regular workload audits are able to review the relationship between patterns of demand and provision, including their appointment systems, their use of telephone communications with patients and their use of all clinical and ancillary staff. These practices seem able to develop the capacity to respond more flexibly.

For most practices, however, activities of this kind have only recently been introduced, stimulated by GPs and practice managers who see organization and its management as a means of enabling everyone in the practice to work more effectively in the interests of patient care and of their own health and enjoyment[1]. Such activities will need to become more widespread as a result of the government's policies in relation to disease prevention and health promotion, the Patient's Charter and complaints procedures, and its determination to see a 'strategic shift' from secondary to primary care.

Some GPs fear that such policies promote a 'practice' rather than 'practitioner' model of care, putting at risk the values of personal continuity of care which underpin the traditional practitioner model[2]. While others challenge this assumption[1], a growing emphasis on the practice as the unit of primary care provision challenges traditional dividing lines between clinical and managerial work. The work of practice managers, secretaries, records clerks and receptionists increasingly includes that of developing and implementing policies and guidelines for health promotion, disease prevention and the management of chronic illness, while the work of clinicians is increasingly influenced by the organization of practice time, space, people, information and equipment.

Increasingly, practice managers draft the practice leaflet, the annual report and the business or practice development plan, and need to understand the clinical activity of the practice in order to do so.

Historically, however, many GPs appointed their first managers out of a need to relieve themselves of some of the day-to-day demands of co-ordinating and supervising a growing band of non-clinical and mainly part-time staff, and of processing increasing amounts of paperwork[3-5].

By the late 1980s 'practice administration' loomed large in studies of GP stress, yet despite growing pressures, many partnerships displayed considerable ambivalence in appointing a manager. Management as a body of knowledge and competence was ignored or dismissed by most GPs for whom it meant bureaucracy, hierarchies and control. Many GPs played safe by promoting senior receptionists or secretaries. Appointments were made without job descriptions and employment contracts, and with little realization of the support and development required by the appointees.

As practices grew in size and complexity during the 1970s, more interest was shown in the development and description of their management. Significantly, the first textbook, although subtitled *A Manual of Practice Management*, was written by four GPs and contains no reference to practice managers[6]. Five years later, what was to prove the major text of the eighties was co-authored by a practice manager and addressed predominantly to the 'new profession' of practice management[7]. This was revised in 1989 and was followed by a spate of books on both practice management *and* the practice manager. Two publishing houses also saw fit to publish practice management literature in loose-leaf binder form, enabling subscribers to keep pace with this burgeoning field[8, 9].

While the majority of managers continued to be appointed from within, the 1990 Contract and GP fundholding provoked many GPs to review their organizations. Consequently, an increasing number of practice managers were recruited from outside general practice, and some of them were men.

Perceptions of the management function by general practitioners and practice managers

This book is based on workshops held during the autumn and winter of 1993/4. At that time, the mood of both GPs and practice managers varied considerably. Some GPs and managers were anxious about the future and their capacity to survive in it; some GPs were provoked by the management focus of the workshops to express profound anger and hostility towards the government's policies and its style of implementing them, and found it difficult to shift their position.

Other GPs and managers, while questioning the adequacy of resources to fund the shift from secondary to primary care, were reasonably confident that they would survive, and even thrive, in the future.

The feelings of both GPs and practice managers related in part to their conceptions of the management function in practice-based primary care. When asked to define this and its distribution within their practices, GPs and practice managers listed such items as finance, staffing, information, premises and equipment, communications, and liaison with the FHSA or health commission.

Whereas items on their lists were similar, groups interpreted them differently. In most groups, each item tended to be interpreted operationally, in terms of those systems and working practices needed to ensure 'the smooth running of the practice'. In some groups, items were also interpreted strategically, as activities necessary to ensure the practice's survival in a rapidly and often unpredictably changing environment.

Typically, the more strategic view came from GPs and practice managers in the larger and the fundholding practices. Many of the smaller practices found it difficult to think of the management function in strategic terms. While some listed 'planning', few displayed a real grasp of the overall interconnection and strategic relevance of individual items such as premises, staffing, finance and information. It was a practice manager from a larger practice who said 'premises are crucial to your whole business strategy and will in part determine what you can and cannot do in the future'.

Similarly, in discussing finance and staff, many of the smaller practices defined these functions in purely administrative terms as 'doing the books' and 'supervising and co-ordinating staff'. Those from larger practices conceived 'finance' and 'staff' as major resources in the practice which linked activity, cost and income, and which through 'proactive' management could ensure that the practice not only survived but thrived in the future. These practices tended to include the partners under 'staff' or 'staffing', analysing the current age, gender and interest mix, how this was serving the needs of the practice now and how it might need to change in the future.

Practices also differed in the mental time frames within which they managed. Larger practices took a longer view and acknowledged that only with effective and efficient management could they meet the medium and longer term future with confidence. Larger practices have usually undergone significant organizational change as they have grown, which may have made them more aware of the need to manage their organizations through time.

In general, the larger the practice, the more the GPs left the day-to-day operational management functions to the practice manager, but this was not always the case. Nor did these GPs always recognize and accept that they themselves, as partners and owners of the business, needed to give strategic direction to the practice.

The delegation of operational management is more probable in the larger practices, because there is recognizably an organization that includes but is, in a sense, external to the GPs themselves as individuals – a situation which GPs in small practices, especially single-handed ones, view with real distaste. One such GP believed that GPs in practices of one or two partners and those in practices of over six were radically different as people. He did not think that he, a single-hander, could ever work in a large practice; it was as if, for him, it would not be 'general practice' in some core sense of the term.

In a single-handed practice, the GP *is* his (or her) organization. The patients are 'his', as are the staff. 'Management', if that is the appropriate term, is the management of one person's clinical practice. If the GP appoints a practice manager, the person usually functions as an administrator and remains embedded within the staff, in the sense of covering for them in absence, but also occupying a staff role such as that of secretary. It is also significant that workshop practice managers who were married to their GPs came exclusively from single-handed practices.

As the number of doctors increases, the number of staff and the size of the building typically increase. While patients might continue to see their own doctor most of the time, there will be occasions when they see another, and they will certainly interact with staff who work for all the doctors. The GPs will typically hire someone they call a practice manager to manage 'the practice', an organization that has now come clearly into being but which apparently does not include them; for GPs tend not to assume that the practice manager will manage them. The practice manager may not manage the practice nurse either, for at this stage the GPs maintain a sharp dividing line between what is considered clinical and what is considered administrative.

Some GPs in the medium-sized practices of three to five partners were both confused and ambivalent about 'management'. They avoided using the term, preferring that of 'administration'. In these practices, practice managers vary more in the way their role is defined, their backgrounds and their own orientation to their role than in the very small, the large and the fundholding practices.

As the number of partners, staff and premises grow the range of services typically increases, as does the range of staff. At this point, 'the practice' has become 'practice-based primary care', following the principle put by one GP: 'Provide to your limits then bring in others'. Fundholding practices in particular have done this over the past four years, but they are not alone.

GPs in practices of six or more partners and in fundholding practices tend to acknowledge that they now have an organization that they are part of in two senses: first, as directors rather than managers, belonging to that group in the organization that must define policy and give a directional steer; second, as doctors who must be held accountable to the practice manager for the organizational aspects of their work, if the policies they agreed as directors are to be implemented effectively.

Not all GPs in large practices translate this acknowledgement into behaviour, but increasingly they recognize that they now work in an organization that is not wholly theirs, in the psychological sense. It is not 'my practice' but 'the practice' and, if it is managed well, the organization can offer GPs much relief from the stress of trying to do everything – of trying to be both clinician and operational manager.

Many GPs still doubt that effective management can reduce their stress, because they are so afraid of losing control. Their perceived loss of control over their own terms and conditions of service at national level appears to have intensified their need to control at practice level. Their sense of stress is compounded by their realization that if they are to regain any sense of control *outside* the practice at the local level, particularly in view of the possibility of localized GP contracts in the future, they need to form positive and proactive links with other practices. This becomes yet another demand on their time, so that the only way it can realistically be achieved is to relinquish some of the control of their own practices, particularly operational aspects.

Factors influencing perceptions of the management function

While practice size appeared to be a major determinant of the way the management function was both perceived and distributed, some small practices were more strategic and some larger practices less so in their approach. These 'exceptions' could usually be attributed to the previous experience, education, interest and orientation of either or both the GP and practice manager. In the past few years some GPs, even in smaller and medium-sized practices, have developed a real interest in their practices as organizations and in their management.

Some of them have developed their interest in the subject of management so far as to attend courses, and even MBA (Master of Business Administration) programmes. Some practice managers in these practices have also developed themselves as managers, attending courses and learning more about management generally, and not just practice management. Some of these practices also recruited practice managers from outside general practice, some of whom challenged and changed their GPs' existing perceptions of management and its appropriate distribution within the practice. Others have been influenced by their use of management consultants, either through arrangements with their health commissions or privately.

In one county in particular, two components of the health commission's primary care development programme have catalysed some of the practices with two to four partners. One is the practice health planning programme in which practices wishing to extend their services, their staff, their premises, or all of these, are asked to write a health plan and are offered the services of a management consultant to help them do this. The other is the Senior Manager Programme through which a practice which wishes to appoint a manager is enabled to recruit on a higher pay scale than would normally apply to their size of practice, providing they agree to include certain components in the job description and to consider the manager a non-equity partner.

The scheme enables the Commission's Assistant Primary Care Manager to engage the partners in full discussion of why they want a manager and how they wish to distribute the management function within the practice. Smaller practices were able to make practice manager appointments that were atypical for their size and there was one appointee who manages two practices of two partners each.

Practice manager job descriptions

Practice manager job descriptions are one indicator of the way in which GPs perceive the management function and its distribution within the practice. They are usually the product of a process in which the partners discuss their need for a manager, although they are also influenced by what the GPs have read, by specimen job descriptions offered on courses or in practice management textbooks, and by FHSAs or health commissions. Some of them are also the product of negotiations between the GPs and the practice manager after appointment, and may be revised over the years.

Job descriptions of practice managers attending the workshops varied in length, content and style – from one of half a sheet of A4 which listed five operational management tasks in almost the same number of lines, to one of five pages, which left no room for doubt as to what the post entailed.

Many comprised lists of regulation-driven tasks which conveyed no sense of the organization's values or culture. These descriptions typically made no reference to the clinical organization of the practice. Most were organized under headings such as:

- major duties and responsibilities

- staff management, training and development

- practice administration

- premises and administration

- non-clinical patient welfare

- financial administration.

It would not be wise to make too much of the wording of these documents, but their use of the terms 'management' and 'administration' is revealing. Whereas 'staff' could be managed by the practice manager, 'the practice' and 'finance' were confined to 'administration' by the manager.

Some practices now recognize that the practice manager works on the boundary between organizational and clinical activity. One job description contained as the job's purpose the words:

> 'to provide executive and administrative support to the partners in managing the non-clinical functions of the practice.'

Whereas the main duties and responsibilities included:

> 'audit/quality assurance and non-clinical patient welfare (complaints and suggestions), and the patient liaison group.'

More unusual was a draft performance contract for a senior manager in Dorset which indicated much more responsibility for managing the clinical/organizational interface:

- participate in initial meetings to plan the health plan

- prepare management processes required for planning the health plan

- prepare an audit system required to run Band 3 Health Promotion

- establish asthma and diabetic monitoring system by end November.

Deadlines were attached to several tasks in this job description, performance against which would determine this manager's performance-related pay.

More remarkable in this job description was the item:

> 'review current management situation of attached staff and advise on their next service level agreements (April 1994 target date) and ensure practice fulfils patients' needs – analyse practice population's needs in line with health service requirements by October 1993. Prepare a Patient's Charter.'

This manager was given the task of reviewing *all* aspects of this practice's organization. These tasks in the job description were mainly strategic. No items referred to claims, records and premises. The document described a general management role, and in that sense was similar to a description from another practice of a post entitled business and development manager. The purpose of this job was:

'to enable the development of practice-based multi-disciplinary services delivered by primary health care staff working
as a team in response to assessed local health needs and to
the financial benefit of the practice.'

Areas of prime responsibility included:

- assessment of local health needs

- planning for service development to respond to health
  needs

- identification of practice strengths and weaknesses.

These job descriptions were clearly 'formalities' for some practices rather than working documents, and some were out of
date. Those written in the past year or so demonstrated newer
thinking especially those for incoming senior managers under
one county's special scheme.

Very few specified any 'results' or indicators of effective
performance, although one fundholding practice stated that
evidence of successful practice management would be found
in:

- high patient satisfaction with the services provided and
  therefore a large list size

- an environment in which the doctors can use their time as
  efficiently as possible

- highly trained and motivated staff members with good
  morale

- full realization of the financial potential of the practice.

This document had been updated to take account of fundholding and referred to the practice manager's need to delegate to
a fund/systems manager, for which post a detailed job description was attached. In all, both descriptions amounted to six
single-spaced A4 sides which conveyed much careful thought.

In the more managerially aware practices, managers are
increasingly being expected to:

'promote the development of the practice-based multi-disciplinary services delivered by primary health care staff working as a team to provide for local health needs. The practice manager will be expected to work closely with the partners as a team to develop, initiate and orchestrate existing and new areas of primary health care and development.'

The role described here is that being performed by some practice managers and aspired to by some others. It is genuinely managerial in that it is about managing change. It tests the manager's capacity for leadership and their capacity to develop leadership in others. As such it is different from other descriptions which list solely the tasks required 'to ensure the smooth running of the practice'. It also conveys that clinical and non-clinical areas of the practice's work are seen as a unified whole. The development of *services* and of primary health *care* is firmly part of the brief.

'The smooth running of the practice'

This phrase occurred repeatedly in job descriptions and in all workshop discussions of the management function in general practice. Its importance must be recognized in order to ensure that effective and efficient *operational* management and administration are not devalued.

General management entered the NHS in 1993 as a result of the Griffiths' review of NHS management[10]. Since that time the models and methods of business management have been imposed on the management of public services, challenging the traditional models and methods of both professionalism and public administration[11,12]. NHS administrators, as they were called at the time, saw the writing on the wall and changed the name of their professional association from the Institute of Health Service Administrators to the Institute of Health Services Management. The National Administrative Training Scheme became first the National Management Training Scheme and subsequently the General Management Training Scheme.

It was assumed that administrators were those who created and sustained smooth running working environments for others, whether these were politicians or doctors. They did not *lead*, nor did they manage change or give strategic direction. Strategic management, in contrast, was considered 'sexy', presumably a reference to the aphrodisiac nature of power. The subsequent introduction of 'the internal market'[13] with its purchaser–provider split, further polarized administration and management in the NHS.

For most of the 1980s these changes bypassed practice-based primary care, although they influenced Community Units and created pressures on their staffs that were ill-understood by GPs. When general management finally entered the Family Practitioner Committees (FPCs) in 1989, and only 50% of their former 'administrators' were successful in their applications for FHSA general manager posts, GPs began to feel the winds of change. The new FHSAs, which replaced the FPCs, were given a more 'managerial' remit, within the constraints imposed by a national GP contract.

As practices increasingly experience pressures to become 'more strategic' and 'more managerial', why is it that they place such emphasis on 'the smooth running of the practice'? As 'the front line of the NHS'[14], to which members of the public have unlimited access free at the point of use, general practice is confronted with anxiety and distress, anger and despair, and many other of life's deepest emotions. All staff, but particularly those in contact with patients and their carers, have to draw a fine line between being empathic and finding themselves overwhelmed by the intensity of others' emotions.

This is the key difference between provider and purchaser organizations, and is the hallmark of human service organizations[15]. Consequently, the self of the individual provider is part of the diagnostic and therapeutic process. In these organizations, a major function of the organization itself is to contain the anxiety not only of its patients or clients but of those who work with them[16-18].

Providing, therefore, that 'the smooth running of the practice' is flexibly rather than rigidly interpreted, it enables the practice to act as just such a container. It fails to do this, however, if it inhibits the organization from also developing the capacity to anticipate and respond constructively to inevitable environmental change. Like individuals, organizations sometimes prefer to deal with their anxiety through adherence to defensive routines[17, 19], which simply exacerbate their inability to come to terms with reality.

The strains on practice-based primary care are particularly acute because of the ambiguous and essentially 'messy' nature of what many patients bring to their GPs[20]. Patients present GPs with signs of biological, psychological and social disturbance which are difficult to disentangle; the source of 'the problem' and its resolution may not lie with the patient; and some patients who have major disease may feel 'well', whereas others who have no disease may feel 'ill'.

The more unpredictable the demand, the more 'messy' the presentation of the problem or problems and the more potentially overwhelming the patient's emotions, the greater the need for a 'smooth running' organizational environment. The development and maintenance of good administrative systems in general practice are consequently imperative. A practice may be superb at strategic planning, but if it cannot anticipate, plan for and monitor the impact of that planning on the day-to-day running of the practice, its organizational and individual stress levels may increase rather than decrease. Some practices are now learning that both effective operational and strategic management are necessary.

Not all practice managers in the workshops wanted a strategic managerial role; neither would all GPs wish to see a non-doctor occupy such a role. The next two chapters identify the factors that had shaped the roles of the practice managers participating in the workshops.

The practice manager role $\boxed{3}$

The practice manager role and practice size

In the smaller practices, the practice manager tends, although not always, to have been promoted from within. The practice manager role also tends to remain embedded in other roles such as those of secretary or senior receptionist. The smaller the practice, the more practice managers find that finances are very tightly controlled by the GPs. Typically, managers are not given a budget to manage and 'have to ask for everything'. The type of involvement practice managers have in 'finance' is one of the major indicators of whether they are truly the managers of the practice or simply office supervisors, senior clerks, book-keepers, and building caretakers – or what has been termed housewives or housekeepers[3,21]. Some practice managers 'do the books', yet are unaware of the doctors' drawings and would certainly not be present at the partners' meetings with their accountant.

In smaller practices, some GPs deliberately continue to employ practice administrators rather than practice managers, preferring to perform operational management work themselves, especially if this involves any risk that money might be lost or not maximized. This was a criterion for one GP of what he would and would not delegate, yet most practice managers worth their salt enhance their practice's income during their first year. In view of some GPs' reluctance to delegate day-to-day management, many GPs in smaller and some medium-sized practices are not developing their views of the future nor any strategy to help them deal with it.

One outstanding exception was a single-handed GP who was trying to bring small practices together for multiple bulk purchasing. Some managers are also trying to promote change, but as many remain embedded within the staff group there is neither the time nor the inclination to think strategically. Typically these managers have undergone little of the type of management education or development that would promote strategic thinking.

This must concern the new health authorities which are being charged to promote a primary-care-led NHS. It is so easy for practice managers as well as GPs to become bogged down in operational management, particularly when new government policies increase the paper-driven routines required to relate work done to payments received. Many GPs are dependent upon their practice managers to catalyse their thinking about the practice as an organization in a changing environment, yet practice managers in some of these practices would neither wish nor be able to do this effectively.

While workshop group numbers were small and generalizations therefore hazardous, it seemed that practices of three or four partners were particularly prone to tensions between GPs and practice managers surrounding the definition of the practice manager's role. Many GPs in these practices were concerned about the capacity of general practice as they know it and like it. Their own sense of pressure is easily projected on to the practice manager.

Typically, they did not bring in practice managers from outside, but are now beginning to wonder whether the practice managers they appointed from inside are capable of the kind of management they now believe to be necessary. Their grasp of this kind of management, however, is not clear. In discussing it, magical expectations were voiced of a new kind of person who would come in and turn the practice around, obviating the necessity for the GPs themselves to change their own orientations and behaviours. Alternatively, when they recruited practice managers from outside, these GPs sometimes got more than they bargained for in someone who wished to manage more than the GPs were willing to give them.

In the larger practices the distribution of management functions is clearer. In most of these, GPs make the policy or set the standard, often with the full involvement of the practice manager who then develops systems to ensure their implementation. As one practice manager in a fundholding practice said:

> 'our core philosophy is that formulation of policy is done by the GPs, and day-to-day management by the practice manager. The partners give me standards like appointment the same day, scripts the same day, and I implement them.'

The role of practice manager develops with increasing size and differentiation within the practice. As one practice manager said:

> 'the number of pots on the boil increases, and we have to keep them bubbling and co-ordinate them all. We keep the whole practice together, we co-ordinate everyone.'

Another said that part of her role was to promote 'the welfare' of the practice and everyone in it, from GPs through all staff, clinical and clerical, and patients. This was a practice of 14 partners with well over 20 000 patients and three premises.

Once practices reach this size, 'sections' and 'section heads' begin to appear. Consequently, the need for the practice manager, and not just the GPs, to delegate emerges. One practice manager was aware that 'the team' was becoming a much bigger concept; that the practice manager needed to think about how best to encourage teams to manage themselves; and how best to help all staff manage change.

In fundholding practices there are signs that practice managers have grown not just as a result of the additional work and the recognition that this made organization and management imperative, but through the close mutual learning relationship between the manager and the leading fundholding GP. While this relationship originates in the organization development needs of the practice, rather than the management development needs of the two individuals, it has provided an opportunity for the two individuals to share practice-based management learning.

The development opportunity has been even greater where this pair have together attended regular monthly meetings of fundholding practices' groups, and where managers of such practices have their own monthly meetings. Such developments have pulled these managers more firmly into 'the board' level of the practice.

In summary, in very small practices the manager in some cases remains embedded within the staff group, rarely influencing the future direction of the practice, unless she is married to the doctor; in medium-sized practices the manager lies between the staff and the GPs in what can be a quite isolated role; in much larger, and particularly in fundholding practices, the manager becomes fully part of the policy and strategy determining group. There are exceptions in each practice size category, but the underlying pattern is there.

From multi-premise to multi-practice provider units?

In the practices of over six partners and of fundholders, there were several examples of very large practices indeed, with over 20 000 patients and over a dozen partners, offering services from three or four sites. Two of these had brought in practice managers from outside, one from the armed services and one from the city-based operations of one of the big clearing banks. Typically, in arrangements of this kind, someone else functions as the manager or administrator of day-to-day operations in each surgery, in a role similar to that of the traditional practice manager of the 1970s and early 1980s.

The task for the incoming manager, whose role approximates that of a general manager elsewhere, is then quite complex. 'The practice' as a business is experienced at a level of abstraction that is not present in the smaller, single surgery organization. Different surgeries may be mini-organizations in their own right, with their own practice populations and their own 'groups' of GPs and primary care teams. Although the partnership is officially the employer, the staff at each surgery may identify with that organization particularly when it is referred to as 'the practice' locally and may have its own name.

GPs in such arrangements may also meet together only as a business partnership, if their clinical practice is confined to one particular surgery apart from on-call rotas and cover for holidays and study leave. Fundholding tends to break down this degree of separation and demand the development of single policies and clinical practices across the organization, for example in prescribing and referrals because these influence the business side of the practice. Several GPs and practice managers referred to the need to develop greater corporate identity in their organizations, an issue faced particularly by large, multi-site practices.

More research is needed into the organizational and managerial challenges faced by multi-site practices. Their managers, in particular, could identify some of the advantages and disadvantages of employing one manager to manage more than one practice, a potential future development raised in these workshops, particularly in relation to small practices wishing to come together. Such managers are able to draw useful comparisons between practices in the amount of resource they use in support of different aspects of the management function and the respective outcomes or outputs from that resource.

Practice manager recruitment and development

GPs tend to get the practice managers they deserve. They find it difficult to define the work they want a practice manager to do, and the work they themselves will need to do if the person entering the post is to be effective. Some GPs are living with the results of their own lack of recruitment skills, to the detriment of themselves, the practice manager and the practice.

The more GPs think about management, the more they realize they do not know. As one GP concluded:

> 'I need to know whether my manager is any good. If *we* don't know about management, how do we know whether our managers are any good?'

This was said after the fact of the manager's recruitment. Did the GPs at the time of recruitment know what they were looking for, or if they did, did they know how to ensure that they got it?

In view of the growing importance of the practice manager role inside the practice and in developing the practice's relationship with its patient population and with the new health authorities, these bodies could usefully offer help to practices who are thinking through and trying to make such appointments. Some GPs in our workshops would be suspicious of too close involvement by health authority managers, whereas others would welcome this, but the provision of booklets, distance learning materials[22,23], consultancy or workshops would probably be acceptable to most practices. It is in the interests of health commissions to make this kind of help available, as the practice manager role is pivotal in the development of more effective and efficient practice-based primary care.

At present practice managers could do a great deal more as change agents within the practices in which they work. Some of those who were promoted from within the practice have been content to remain in a supervisory and administrative role. Others, stimulated by the developments of the past few years, have grown with the practice and acted as catalysts, urging their GPs to take a more strategic view of the practice in its environment. A close working relationship with one or more GPs who are taking managerial responsibilities within the partnership appears to be critical in enabling the manager to work in this way.

A minority of GPs in the workshops felt that in order to face a threatening future, they might need a different kind of manager from the one they have now. They do not appear to consider that their managers, with help, might develop into the different kind of manager they feel they need. They would be unsure how to identify their managers' development needs, and would have little idea how and by whom these might be met.

GPs and practice managers in those practices which are expanding in size and complexity need to discuss honestly the needs of the practice as they perceive them, and the current capacity, competence and motivation of the existing practice manager. Given the capacity to develop in response to practice changes and the motivation to go on doing so, these practice managers need the educational and development opportunities to be able to grow in line with the changing practice manager role.

The new health authorities have a potentially large and helpful role to play here, but need to manage it sensitively. There is also a need for a national strategy for practice management development that will accommodate the different needs of practice managers and GPs.

Recruitment from outside

A challenge to GPs' perceptions of their organizations and the need for better management within them has come from the appointment of practice managers from outside general practice. These recruits, particularly those from commercial organizations, were surprised by what they perceived to be the low level of development of the business side of the practice. One identified the practice manager role to be that of developing 'the business', for 'some GPs are losing money as the ways of making money are decreasing'. He was probably referring here to the new health promotion arrangements of 1993.

These practice managers also found bizarre the financial management arrangements in general practice compared to those they had seen elsewhere. Managers entering general practice from both the public and private sectors were surprised by the secrecy surrounding doctors' drawings, and the fact that 'profits' were not seen as organizational profits to be reinvested in the business nor used to pay higher salaries or bonuses to staff, but as doctors' earnings to be translated into higher drawings or higher pension contributions for the doctors.

They found remarkable the lack of pensions for staff, including managers, in general practice in view of the profits going into GP pensions. Some had negotiated pensions with their employers on entering the practice, but as yet pensions for staff are not widespread.

Historically, GPs were protected from the link between pay and conditions and quality of staff, for they were able to offer local employment in small, family-like organizations with flexible hours. Female employees who were attracted by these features were so grateful for them that they did not demand those other conditions that were considered normal in larger, more formalized organizations.

Until the 1990s this did not matter unduly, but in view of the current pressure on practices to develop the organizational context of their clinical work and to manage more proactively the boundary between the practice and the outside world, practices will need to review the current link between the conditions they offer and the staff they are able to recruit. Many practices have already begun to do this.

Underlying this issue is the unique arrangement whereby independent contractors are legally the employers of considerable numbers of people whose salaries are funded largely by the Exchequer. As an 'expense', staff salaries and conditions are also an issue for negotiators of the national GP contract and for the authorities which manage that contract.

Many GPs complain that they cannot pay higher salaries for practice managers, because their FHSAs will not 'allow' them to do so. If they wish to effect a strategic shift from secondary to primary care, the new health authorities might need to consider more direct means of influencing the quality of practice managers beyond those of funding management development opportunities for them. They might also need to consider factors in addition to practice size in reviewing their criteria for reimbursement of practice manager salaries.

The possibility of practice managers entering into profit sharing agreements with partners was raised in the workshops, and one partnership and an incoming manager were discussing the possibility of performance-related pay.

Practice managers from outside also tend to take a different view of patients than those who have grown from within the practice. They find it easy to see patients as a population, because they tend to see them as a potential 'market' in the soft sense of the term, and as 'customers' or 'consumers' rather than patients. This difference was less marked in the larger practices, whose internally promoted managers are more likely to have attended management courses which have given them a broader business management perspective.

Many practice managers who have grown from within the practice from secretarial, reception or nursing positions identify with 'their' GPs and were quite shocked by some of the observations made by newcomers. Some of this identification by established managers relates to their recognition of the special nature of health care organizations, to which people as patients bring the most intense of life's emotions. As individuals who have grown from within the practice, they have been effectively socialized by 'their' GPs into 'the practitioner model of care'[2]. They often 'administer' the clinical practice of *each*

GP as if he or she were single-handed, with members of staff expected to accommodate to the individual working practices of each GP.

Most of the entrants to practice management from outside general practice were recent appointments. Although they will probably never absorb the culture of general practice as fully as have practice managers who have grown with their practices, they will over the next year or so begin to recognize what makes health care organizations in general, and general practice in particular, 'different'. It would be unfortunate, however, if this acculturation process were so successful as to erase their capacity to be objective. This capacity is needed if general practice is to influence the future direction of health care in this country[24].

General practice as a profession has not been particularly effective in translating its gut level rejection of many of the government's NHS 'reforms' into a sustained, well-constructed critique of the uncritical application of market and consumer terminology to health care. Pratt makes a sustained attempt to do this, but even he wrestles with the risk of polarizing practitioner and practice models of care[2]. The challenge is not to plump for either one or the other (although no doubt some GPs and some practices will do so), but to integrate the two. More research is needed to discover whether such integration is possible and practicable and, if so, then to identify its prerequisites.

The demographics and economics of health care make it inevitable that clinical freedom within publicly funded health care systems will be constrained, and re-granted only in return for greater and more specific accountability.

The recent entry of some managers from the business world into general practice may, at the level of the practice, forge better relations between the small business and professional aspects of general practice that have always to some extent been in tension. The challenge is to render that tension creative so that clinicians and managers feel empowered rather than disempowered by it. Some practices are now managing this tension much more creatively than they have in the past.

Without exception, they are marked by their GPs' recognition that *management* is, like general practice, a discipline in its own right and that the manager must be given the organizational space to apply it. This is not to say that GPs in these practices take a hands-off approach to management and to their managers. Rather, *they work with their managers to clarify those aspects of management that are best addressed by the GPs as directors and as clinicians and those that are best addressed by the manager.*

In contrast, some GPs are now so threatened by developments in the NHS that they feel they must 'reclaim' the management of their own practices. Ideally, this would mean that as partners they would take the time to review the management function and its current distribution against their perceptions of future demands. Ideally, they would also involve their practice managers and staff in this vital activity. Consequently, they should be able to clarify what as GPs they must manage and what they can safely delegate.

It would be wasteful and stressful if, in their anxiety, they simply hung on to or grabbed back the day-to-day management of the practice.

Gender issues in practice management

The entry into practice management of retired armed services personnel, or early retirees from financial institutions such as banks and building societies, has raised for female practice managers some painful gender issues in practice management.

When asked why they were appointing people, usually men, from these backgrounds, some GPs replied that these new recruits had 'good man management skills' (sic) and that because they already had pensions, they were attractively affordable. Other reasons were: these men were attracted by

stability and structure, and by a culture of loyalty, which typified general practice; their age and proven previous career
brought advantages to the practice; service personnel were also
usually aware of the processes of funding in public organizations.

The results of these appointments vary, depending on the
motivation of the GPs and the incoming manager. Structure
and order may appear to replace chaos; what is not clear is
whether the practice develops a greater capacity to relate more
intelligently and assertively to its environment, and to manage
change actively rather than passively. The armed services, and
indeed the banks, can be as blind as general practice to
unpalatable external realities. Consequently, there is a risk that
some appointees may collude with their practices' failure to
develop those policies and strategies that will take them
through the 1990s.

For managers who have never worked in general practice,
the scale of the transition required is considerable. Just as
practice managers who have come up through the practice
need the opportunity to develop knowledge and skills in business management, those who come into practice management
from outside need an opportunity to learn about the nature
of general practice, of the NHS, and of 'the health care
industry'.

Some GPs are easily impressed by managers who enter
general practice from established managerial careers outside,
particularly when they are male. Consequently, they tend to
underestimate these managers' transition needs. This is not an
argument for 'socializing' new recruits into practice management in such a way that they over-identify with GPs, thereby
neutralizing their capacity to challenge existing structures and
processes within the practice, but induction is necessary.

When established male managers from the services, the
banks or any other sector are brought in from outside, they
may be given an unchallenged managerial role within the
practice. When female external appointees are introduced,
their role may remain ambiguous while the previous incumbent serves out her time until retirement. This difficult situa-

tion is also experienced by practice staff who undertake management training and are subsequently promoted over an existing manager.

Most practice managers in smaller practices continue to be promoted from within. They frequently continue to carry secretarial responsibilities, and may be expected to 'help out on reception'. This does not help the woman, and it is usually a woman, in her transition into a managerial role. One of the managers in the workshops was given the title 'practice manageress, so as not to upset the girls'. Avoidance of the status and authority shifts implied in such pseudo-promotions remains common. Some women are sufficiently ambivalent about their promotion that they collude in the avoidance, thereby sabotaging the possibility of needed organizational change.

Practice managers in the smaller practices also found it difficult to enter the finance and information technology components of the management function. If they were young and female they were not seen by the GPs to possess these skills. Several women practice managers voiced doubts about their competence in these areas, in common with many women who enter management jobs from traditionally female occupations. The achievements of internally promoted women practice managers in many fundholding practices, however, testifies to their capacity to become competent and confident in these areas – given the necessity to do so, support from a lead GP and availability of training.

Many female practice managers coming through the practice ranks continue, however, to experience difficulties in their transition. It is never easy for those who are promoted within organizations to modify the perceptions of those with whom they worked in their former roles.

It is particularly difficult for women who are promoted into management roles, for in so doing they may move from an occupational role associated with females (nurse, receptionist, secretary) into one associated predominantly with males. Early practice manager roles were similar to those of office supervisors or administrative assistants, which were considered appropriate for women. Some GPs *and* practice managers have colluded in maintaining such a concept of the practice manager, particularly in smaller practices.

'Practice management' remains as yet a 'gendered' occupation. A recent survey of 503 practice managers conducted by the Institute of Health Services Management contained only 19% male respondents. This percentage probably overestimates the numbers of male practice managers, as the survey population comprised those practice managers who responded to a questionnaire circulated in the journal *Practice Manager*. Consequently, they were managers who were sufficiently interested in their work and occupation to read the journal, and to read and respond to the questionnaire. (*See* Appendix 1 for further comment on this survey.)

In the workshops, particularly those for the larger and fundholding practices, several women practice managers had entered general practice from established careers outside, for example from NHS management, the clearing banks, the civil service, and so on. They, like some of their male counterparts, brought new perspectives. They tend to lead from behind, however, just as do female practice managers who have established themselves over years within the same practice. As a generalization which does not always hold true, GPs seem more willing to accept and indeed expect that incoming male practice managers will lead from the front.

Few female practice managers developed their capacities by moving between practices. Those who did so testified to its value in developing them as managers, as did those few GPs who had experienced more than one practice. Most female practice managers have husbands and families and may as a result be required, or prefer, to settle in an area for some time. Practice managers who come up through the ranks in general practice also absorb its culture of loyalty.

This does not mean that female practice managers' learning and development is confined to the one practice in which they work. Practice managers in the workshops related with increasing frequency to the health commission and its managers, a development welcomed by some GPs but met with anxiety by others. They also related with increasing frequency to practice managers in other practices through devices like fundholding manager groups, locality groups of practice managers and other types of learning groups which are increasingly fostered by health commissions and the Association of Managers in General Practice (AMGP).

In due course, this might lead to more movement of managers across practices in the course of their careers. The variety of size and type of organization now presented by modern general practice is beginning to hold out a prospect of a true 'career' in practice management, beginning in a smaller practice and moving to a larger one. It also offers lateral career movement so that if a practice manager in a rapidly growing practice which is also contemplating fundholding does not want to take on a broader range of responsibilities in a larger, more complex practice, she has the opportunity of moving to a smaller one.

The evidence suggests that some women will not want to take on a more demanding role for several reasons – including age, family responsibilities which include not only children but aged parents, or simply personal preference. In many practices which are increasing in size and complexity there is often the possibility of staying in the practice, as someone else is brought in at a more senior level, but this has implications for the incumbent manager, GPs and staff, and it may be that the manager prefers a move to a smaller, less complex organization.

The practice manager job title

The comfort of many female practice managers with the title 'practice manager' was apparent when one externally recruited practice manager in a large practice group asserted that in view of the futures participants had postulated, the role would more appropriately be titled 'general manager'. While the only man in the group agreed, most of the other women demurred, distancing themselves from the idea.

One GP who brought in a male manager from the financial services sector had previously employed a female practice manager who had come up through the practice over 20 years. This GP now considers that she was not a manager, but an administrator.

> 'The new man came in and took a totally new view of the practice, much of what he saw he found ridiculous. We agreed that he would be the boss and not the GPs.'

An 'away day' at a local hotel for the two male partners and the incoming manager proved 'so valuable'.

> 'He (the new manager) came up with the model of the GPs and himself as directors of the business, then the manager as manager, and the GPs and staff below.'

This GP's account was viewed with some horror by his GP colleagues in the workshop, but there seemed little doubt that the partners had given their manager 'permission' to do what was necessary to ensure that policies decided at 'board' level by the GPs and manager were implemented by the GPs when working as doctors. He also felt that the presence of the manager had freed up the partners' relationship.

The impact on the partnership of these incoming and highly experienced managers from other settings is not unlike that of a management consultant. They bring in an approach that is radically new to GPs, and if they do it in a subtle and not overbearing way, the GPs may be readily impressed, recognizing that this person has a body of knowledge and skill that is not possessed by doctors. If incoming managers are able to convey the advantages they can bring to practices as businesses and to GPs as clinicians, then GPs are readier to delegate, particularly if as in this case, the manager helps them develop keen performance criteria against which he can be measured.

Incoming male managers tend not to hesitate to 'assert' their authority of expertise, which is in turn boosted by the GPs' perceptions of their former careers as senior managers in household name financial institutions such as banks or building societies. Business-oriented GPs are easily captured by this; several female managers identified these 'unbroken managerial careers' as a major competitive advantage for male managers to GPs who wish to effect major change in their practices. The less clear GPs are about the managerial requirements of their own organizations, the more reassured they may be by a manager's 'unbroken managerial career' elsewhere and by his managerial self-confidence at interview.

Research is urgently needed into the prerequisites of effective GP–practice manager relationships, with particular focus on gender issues. The workshops contained some relatively new relationships, which may have been enjoying a kind of 'honeymoon' effect. The male manager described above had also impressed his GPs by conducting a review not only of what the practice nurses did, but what the community nurses did. That he should assume the right to cross the traditional boundary between clinical and managerial in the practice and indeed between the practice and the Community Trust suggests that he was assuming managerial control of the whole practice. His GP intimated that he had given the manager explicit authority to do this.

As increasing numbers of women with established managerial careers are also entering practice management, it would be useful to compare their experience with that of the men. Issues of managerial style, and male and female perceptions of what styles are appropriate to male and female managers are involved[25]. One such new entrant woman manager had been told by her GPs that she had been chosen in preference to male applicants because her management style fitted the ethos of their practice.

Women doctors

Gender issues in practice management relate not only to practice managers, but also to female GPs. It is often said by male GPs that female GPs demonstrate little evidence of interest in and commitment to management. Whereas GPs attending our workshops selected themselves to attend and were not therefore necessarily representative, those female GPs who attended, and there were several, were very interested in management. Significantly, they fell predominantly into the very small and the medium-sized practices. Some had chosen single-handed practice because of the increased control it gave them over the kind of general practice medicine they wished to practise and the organization they felt would best support this.

One female single-hander had formed a cluster with another practice in order to become fundholding. She was typical of single-handers who 'fear being left behind'. Like other single-handed female GPs, she saw herself as both GP and practice manager in her own practice and felt that 'management in practice evolved from the personalities who are already there'. Significantly, however, she judged that the other practice's manager was 'extremely good' and that one of the attractions of clustering was that she could tap into that resource.

She was at pains to point out that only the fundholding component of management was 'combined' and that otherwise she maintained her independence. Like other female single-handers she valued this greatly, feeling that it enabled her to make decisions quickly. Formerly, in a group practice, she came away from meetings feeling very frustrated as no decisions were ever made. In contrast, she now 'has my practice meeting in the bath' and if she wants a computer she goes out and gets it.

Like other female single-handers she also felt that women get a bad deal in general practice, not simply in terms of status and pay, but also the type of patients they get. Many women GPs in larger practices attract more than their fair share of gynaecological and of psychosocial problems. In single-handed practice, particularly in a rural area, single-handed women GPs enjoy a wider range of patients.

Several female single-handers seemed loath to delegate and consequently felt overloaded by both clinical and managerial work. One woman doctor, however, was delegating more to her practice manager inside the practice as she attempted to develop outside it a group of GPs who would influence local purchasing.

Some female single-handed GPs seemed to run their practices as they would their families, with little separation of home and work life, although this pattern has always been common to rural, single-handed GPs. One woman GP went home to lunch as a GP and returned in the afternoon 'as a practice manager'. Another had a computer at home, but not in the practice.

These female single-handed GPs also found it difficult or impossible to sack staff, even when it was clear that the staff concerned would not work in ways demanded by changes in primary care organization. Reasons for reluctance or inability to dismiss included personal affection for staff and concern about how dismissal would be perceived by the local community.

Decision making in general practice

Introduction

The bane of most practice managers' lives is the inability of their GPs to take and implement decisions. This inability is widely acknowledged by GPs themselves and is a major source of frustration to them, as well as to their managers.

Several practices represented in the workshops were 'in flight from autocracy'. Previous experience of senior partner dominance, with its associated anger and frustration, has produced in some practices a state of 'dysfunctional democracy'. Many practice managers recognized the state, without sometimes being aware of its root cause, particularly if they had recently entered general practice from another field.

One GP said that in his practice:

> 'one person can block change so we can end up with the lowest common denominator. Is that a strength or a weakness? It depends on whether it's me. But I do perceive it as a weakness.'

Another GP recognized, very insightfully, that 'not making decisions can be misplaced respect for your other partners'.

Alternatively, partnerships may leave decision taking to one of their number who often has the closest relationship with the practice manager. These two, in face of the other GPs' refusal to be involved, may in desperation take vital decisions, only to find that those GPs fail to implement them.

The desire to avoid autocracy has not been accompanied by the competence and skill in managing group process that is necessary if decisions are to be built, taken and implemented. GPs abhor 'unnecessary bureaucracy'. This term is used to describe both excessive paperwork and excessive meetings, yet as practices grow in size and in the range of people (GPs, other health professionals, support staff) working in them, communication can no longer be left to chance, and if key decisions need to be taken and implemented, meetings are inevitable.

One fundholding practice had a range of meetings, each with a clearly delineated function:

- partnership meeting (once per month)

- clinical meeting (once per month)

- fundholding meeting (once per month)

- the practice meeting (8–9 am one weekday/weekly open to all who wish to come)

- 'away' meetings – for partners and practice manager to engage in strategic planning, in developing their capacity to make decisions and to overcome specific problems, e.g. dismissing someone within the team.

Many GPs dread meetings, probably because they have not yet learned to make them productive. Many GPs also continue to be loath to involve practice staff widely in meetings, feeling that this would make meetings difficult to manage and that there would be dangers in involving staff who might not have adequate information and who might want something that was not wanted by the partners.

Many GPs perceive a large gulf between their own and their staff's level of involvement in and commitment to the practice, and for some GPs 'the practice' means the partnership. More practices are now being required to produce practice business or health plans in order to obtain resources. Consequently, they will need to learn that the more people are involved in the early stages of a development, the more ownership they feel of it and the more ready they are to implement it. Many GPs are aware of the strength of this principle in treating their patients, but do not think to apply it in managing their staff.

GPs would tolerate meetings more readily if they were perceived to be productive, if needed decisions were made and subsequently implemented. The capacity to build, take and implement decisions continues to elude too many GP partnerships, by GPs' own admission.

Impact of NHS changes

The 1990 Contract and the introduction of GP fundholding undoubtedly increased the capacity of partnerships to talk through policy developments that would affect their lives and to decide where they stood on them. They then had to decide what to do as a result. Both GPs and practice managers recognized, however, that even when the partners, often with the help of the practice manager, had taken a decision, their willingness to implement it was suspect, particularly when this involved changing their own behaviour as doctors.

Some GPs as well as practice managers also acknowledged continued difficulty in taking important decisions, even in fundholding practices. The introduction of fundholding tested partnerships' capacity to make and implement decisions. It also appears to have broken the mould of dysfunctional democracy which implied that in order to take any decision, whatever its degree of importance, every member of the partnership had to be fully informed and fully involved.

In many fundholding practices, the day-to-day management of this new initiative was undertaken by the GP who had been the strongest advocate of the scheme and by the practice manager or newly-introduced 'fund manager' or 'business manager'. This structure embodied within the practice the principle of delegation, which GPs have traditionally resisted, in both clinical and managerial areas of their work. It also required, as does any delegation within a group, that the other GPs trust those actively managing to exercise discretion in an area of the practice's work for which there were few blueprints, considerable unpredictability and uncertainty, and possibly ambivalence in some of the other partners.

This was a major learning experience for many partnerships, but one from which they have benefited considerably. This capacity to let go and to trust is beginning to extend to other areas.

Some fundholders in the workshops shared the management functions across the partnership, but had often found that individual partners had to check back with the others. Fundholding, as one GP said, 'loosened the string'. He described his organization now as:

> 'a fully managed practice with a lot of delegation, partners who are free of nuts-and-bolts management, with basic assumptions about who was doing what turned into definite rules.'

Their more flexible staffing, prescribing and purchasing budgets provided incentives to manage and develop staff, and to develop agreed clinical policies in relation to prescribing and referral.

Both GPs and practice managers in fundholding practices increasingly perceive the subtle interaction of clinical, fundholding and managerial aspects of the practice. Consequently, they are able to take a much broader view of their organization's activities as a whole. These practices were also among the first to forge much closer relationships with the rest of the NHS, for example with district and regional health authorities as well as with FHSAs.

Because of their role as purchasers they also had to negotiate relationships with local providers (not just consultants) and social services, and with organizations in the private and voluntary sectors. One fundholding practice manager said that liaising with outside agencies had become such a large task since fundholding, that the practice had to delegate it. Now 'lots of people in the practice liaise and the practice manager co-ordinates'. She considered that delegating responsibilities had developed practice staff dramatically, particularly in their understanding of the practice as an organization in the wider NHS environment.

Both GPs and managers in these practices were clear that at least one GP should take a lead role with the manager in fundholding management, because of the need for clinical input into contracting and negotiating.

Fundholders also faced constant changes, such as the introduction of a further range of services which could be purchased from April 1993, with more in the pipeline. Because of the controversy surrounding the scheme both locally and nationally, many fundholding practices recognized their 'shared fate' and locally, regionally and nationally associated quite closely with each other. This enhanced an already sharp sense of empowerment.

Although the workshops provided examples of new, male practice manager appointments from outside the NHS to fundholding practices, there were many more examples of female practice managers who had been with their practices for some years and had demonstrated remarkable capacity and courage in tackling an unprecedented level and rate of change.

Division of management function within the partnership

Within the bigger practices, and particularly within fundholders, partnerships are now becoming happier to experiment with a clear division of managerial function within the partnership. This takes two predominant forms, which may or may not overlap.

One is specialization of the managerial function across the partnership, e.g. one partner (or two) will carry responsibility for financial management, another for staffing, and so on. One practice carried this as far as having specific objectives for each portfolio. The other is the development of 'the executive partner' concept, in which one GP is designated executive partner, either for a specified period of time or for the foreseeable future.

The difference between this role and that of the senior partner lies in there being no assumptions of 'dead (or retired) men's shoes', or 'longest in, next up'. If the role goes to the GP who is acknowledged as most fitted for it, adoption of the executive partner role within a partnership suggests a level of organizational sophistication in a practice. It requires that the partners acknowledge each other's strengths and weaknesses, and give leadership to one of their number – capacities which tend to elude independent professionals.

For practice managers, the executive partner model has considerable attractions. One practice manager working within this model said:

> 'if you don't have an executive partner, you can lose loads of ideas – they are just not filtered and caught.'

The pairing of executive partner and practice manager inherent in this model, however, carries organizational and personal risks.

- Their shared commitment to and enthusiasm for improved management of the practice may result in their running too far ahead of the other partners. The more time the pair spend on management *as a pair* the greater the risk that they will lose touch with where other partners are in their thinking.

- Because of their own lack of interest in management, the other partners may collude with the pair, encouraging them to shoulder the whole managerial burden of the practice. The pair may subsequently be amazed and hurt by the accusation and abuse piled upon them as a result of some decision or action they took in the belief that they had the full support of the rest. Such reactions suggest that the other partners had set boundaries to the extent of the pair's authority which remained tacit rather than explicit.

• Pairing in organizations, as in families and small groups, may provoke envy and jealousy, particularly if the pair appear to have and enjoy something not possessed by others, not least their affection and regard for each other. Practices are not exempt from such primitive reactions.

• As 'a minority of one' who sits on the boundary between the partnership and the staff, the practice manager can feel the need for support within the practice. The demands imposed on practices over the past few years have stretched the capacities of practice managers as much if not more than those of GPs. Consequently, many managers feel the need for guidance, direction and feedback, some of which may be difficult to secure from a group of partners, particularly if they do not function well as a group. As the pair learns to function well as a management unit, the practice manager may direct these needs to the individual GP rather than to the partnership. This in turn creates conditions for a 'special relationship' that may promote greater identification with and loyalty to that GP on the part of the manager. This puts at risk the manager's capacity to catalyse and support the partnership *as a group*.

• GPs are usually attracted to work in the one-to-one situation and to respond to *individual* need. It is therefore easy for the GP to collude in meeting the practice manager's needs and in becoming his or her 'confidante'. Workshop evidence suggests that the support of an individual GP is often crucial in developing the female practice manager's confidence.

Identification of the risks should not deter practices from adopting the executive partner model. Indeed, risk identification is the first step in risk management. The key issue is that of boundaries within the organization. The practice manager occupies a boundary role between the partnership and the staff[26]. Kahn demonstrated many years ago that the occupants of such roles were particularly prone to carry high doses of organizational stress[27].

In appointing an executive partner, the partnership creates a potentially new management unit of that partner and the practice manager, simply because of the amount of time they will spend together focused on the management of the whole organization. The executive partner himself then steps into a boundary role between the partnership and this new management unit. The unit has no legal status in the sense that the partnership and the employed status of the manager are legal entities. It is typically an 'informal' organizational arrangement in most practices, but one with considerable potential consequences for the practice and for the two individuals involved.

Before adopting this model, partnerships need to be as honest as possible about the perceived strengths, weaknesses, opportunities and threats it presents – to the partnership as a group, to its individual members and not least to the practice manager. If the model is adopted, its implementation should be open to regular review particularly in the early stages.

Some practices use the executive partner device but allocate the role in strict rotation for strictly defined time periods. This does not demand the level of trust and 'followership' demanded by allocating the role on 'merit' as judged by other members of the partnership. One fundholding practice had an 'executive group' of three out of eight partners, working with the practice manager.

Some practices which have not developed a managerial structure within the partnership are nevertheless able to build, take and implement what they feel to be necessary decisions. Typically, one partner possesses particularly effective chairmanship skills and there is tacit ageement that he (and it is usually he) exercises these to the benefit of all.

Effective decision taking is also possible in practices in which the partners like each other as people and share a common culture, in particular their assumptions about what is good general practice. Interpersonal affection and regard is a real strength in some partnerships, but if not a rarity, it is certainly not present in many practices.

Not only are partnerships dogged by interpersonal conflicts, but also by radically different definitions of the nature and future of general practice itself. Governmental policy over the past five years has flushed out these differences which previously, in long periods of relatively little change in general practice, could continue unacknowledged as individual GPs continued to function to all intents and purposes as single-handed practitioners while formally being part of a group. Skilled practice managers can catalyse the partnership's capacity to function as an effective group which has important decisions to make if it is to thrive, let alone survive, in the 1990s.

Fundholding has introduced a further feature into partnerships which are trying to develop management structures and processes capable of dealing with a business of growing size and complexity, namely the willingness of partners to grant the leading fundholding partner or the executive partner a number of clinical sessions (typically half days) to devote to the management task.

In view of many partnerships' sensitivity to money issues, and particularly to any perceived inequity in financial arrangements, this testifies to an increasing awareness that modern general practice can be run only from a sound organizational base in which those who manage the organization should be given the time to do so, without this becoming a burdensome 'add on' to clinical work.

Providing there is sufficient awareness of the prerequisites of effective and efficient management of the organization, and high levels of trust and interpersonal regard within the partnership, the executive partner or subgroup arrangement within the partnership can liberate everyone to do what it is they enjoy doing without feeling guilty or put upon.

Without these preconditions, such arrangements may provoke great tension and resentment, born from a sense of exclusion and of becoming 'merely a worker here' by the remaining GPs. Unless these preconditions are met, the portfolio management arrangement which embraces *all* members of the partnership is a safer solution, though the need to liaise with each GP around his portfolio may incur more work for the practice manager. This task and the time it requires may be less onerous than that of mediating in chronic partnership conflict.

By any comparison, the majority of general practices remain very small organizations in which individuals, particularly the GPs, exert great influence on the functional capacity of the whole organization. The alienation of even one GP can, as most practice managers are aware, spoil the whole climate of the practice.

Each practice has to identify, create and develop the particular set of management arrangements that will ensure that it achieves its aims and becomes the kind of practice it wants to be within the various constraints and opportunities offered by current and future health policy. The length of time and the amount of tense and often stressful discussion within partnerships before these arrangements are established cannot be overemphasized – and many practices are a long, long way from this point.

If the direction of the NHS is now to be driven or led by these small organizations which are prone to interpersonal conflict and to uncertainties and insecurities surrounding the appropriate managerial structure they should adopt, much more research will be required into these structures, their origins and their outcomes.

Externally facilitated organization or team development

Many practices described in the workshops had been helped by externally facilitated organization or team development, either by a consultant coming into the practice, or key players in the practice attending a residential workshop.

Organization development offers protected time and space to work on relationships, feelings and processes which inhibit an organization's capacity to build, take and implement decisions. In recent years, many practices have come to value 'away days' as a device for ensuring that they do give time to the strategic management of the practice and to development of their own capacity to act corporately.

'Away days', held outside the practice in particular, also offer protected time and space in which to tackle particularly intractable problems, such as difficult staffing decisions. The day-to-day pressures on general practice are such that frustrations can accumulate around the failure of any one person to perform, whether this be a partner or any member of staff. Because general practices are small organizations, any staffing decision has great consequences for the climate and effectiveness of the practice as a whole. Such decisions may have unfortunate consequences if taken on the run. As one GP who faced just such a problem said, 'the away day offered a useful island in a sea of commotion'.

The most striking example of the success of out-of-practice, residential events was offered by a third wave fundholding practice of five partners. The three-day residential event appeared to have revolutionized the organization of this practice. One of the partners acknowledged that four years ago crisis management dominated the practice, that they had lost one and taken on some new partners, but that from the three-day event 'things had really moved'. They had managed a major extension to premises, total refurbishment, revised their management structure, roles and responsibilities, with each partner overseeing a particular management area. Meetings were reviewed and restructured, and staff were keenly involved in agreeing and implementing direction in the practice.

They were able to make a decision to go fundholding and to develop an appropriate structure and processes for this. The GPs recognized the value of their existing staff and created new and demanding roles for them. The GP spoke enthusiastically and completed his account with the phrase 'we love change'. The practice appears to have created an organization which is capable of containing anxiety and enabling people, through management processes they have themselves created, to feel some confidence that they can manage their future.

The establishment of managerial processes by which management arrangements within a practice can be regularly reviewed against organizational demands will be imperative in ensuring the practice's capacity to survive and thrive in the futures envisaged by GPs and practice managers at the workshops.

Some practices were using the services of management consultants supplied by the health commission in support of the practice health planning process. They found these consultants useful in helping them to adopt an observer's view of their own organizations and of the relationship between the GPs and the practice manager in particular.

Some practices discovered that pressures exerted by policy-driven deadlines had forced them to develop their decision-making capacity. One practice learned from this and began to hold its practice meeting between 8 and 9 am, knowing that it had to end at 9 am when surgery began.

Several of the practices which worked so hard on developing their management arrangements experienced a real sense of achievement. One GP said, 'we have achieved in four years what would normally have taken us eight'.

Although no GPs or practice managers in these workshops used the term 'the learning organization'[28], that is what some, albeit a small minority as yet, had become or were in process of becoming. One GP actually said, 'We're learning'. When asked how they were doing that, he replied:

'through our meetings, through gathering information and
assessing it . . . through our away days . . . all our strategic
thinking is done on these days . . . we must have looked at
our appointment systems 20 times . . . we will re-examine it,
go through it again and again to get it right, get it better.'

Willingness to take the time and trouble to review working
practices on this scale is still rare in general practice. Many GPs
and practice managers in the workshops were unable to find,
or rather to make, that time and space available to themselves.
Those practices which feel overwhelmed by what they experience as unremitting patient and government demands feel
unable to step back and look at how their own behaviours
might contribute to their stress. This in turn reduces the
likelihood that they will develop even the most minimal
managerial arrangements and processes that would begin to
enable them to function more effectively. Meanwhile, their
colleagues who have begun to develop such arrangements and
processes find that their learning and their greater efficiency
release yet more time and space for further review and im-
provement.

The deep antipathy many GPs feel towards 'management',
which for them smacks of bureaucracy, hierarchy and control,
makes them hang on to areas of management which they could
safely delegate. Almost all practice managers in the workshops,
apart from a few in fundholding and very large practices, felt
able to take on more of the management of the practice than
GPs were willing to give them, particularly if the GPs concen-
trated on providing a practice policy framework and strategic
direction.

The more GPs insist on controlling day-to-day, or operational, management of the practice, the less they will provide
the very thing their practice managers need in order to manage well, namely that policy framework and strategic direction.

Clinical and managerial work is most likely to overlap at the
operational level and many GPs especially those in small practices, are adamant that the 'lay' (i.e. non-medical) manager
shall not enter the clinical arena of the practice in any way.

Much of what was previously seen to be 'clinical' care is, however, now the province of the whole practice and not simply the GP. In particular, the management of chronic disease and of health promotion and disease prevention is a practice or primary care team task that needs to be managed if it is to be done effectively and efficiently.

The resistance of some GPs to delegation of management tasks is mirrored by their resistance to delegation of some clinical tasks to other health professionals. GPs, as owners of their own small business, can still choose the work they do and, within limits, the level of support they wish to have to help them do that work. The continuation of relatively isolated single-handed practice and indeed the strong preference for it by many GPs, not least those who have experienced difficulty working in partnerships, is testament to this freedom to choose.

It is also, of course, a testament to the freedom of patients to choose their doctor. Many patients, not only in rural but in inner city areas, are devoted to their single-handed doctors, despite in many cases their lack of both administrative and clinical support staff. For some groups in the population, particularly the elderly and socially isolated, the GP may be the one of the few continuing figures in their lives. The GP may also embody key aspects of their own biography, particularly relationships that are now lost to them through death or separation.

As Marsh and Kaim-Caudle demonstrated some years ago, patients are remarkably tolerant of the pattern of care offered by their GPs and are easily persuaded to accept changes providing their doctor appears to approve of them[29]. Subsequent authors emphasized the importance of planned and careful communication with patients when introducing changes in the pattern of provision, whether through introduction of practice nurses[30], social workers[31] or more broadly across the primary care team[1].

Managers in the new health authorities will need to beware speaking of the preferences of 'the GP' and 'the patient' in the singular. Increasingly, preferences for different organizational models of delivering primary care are being expressed by different *groups* of GPs and different *groups* of patients. Prior to the 1980s, and particularly the 1990s, the dominant model of care was practitioner-centred rather than patient-centred[2]. Over the past 20 years the proportion of single- and two-handed practices has declined in proportion to the rise of practices with over five partners. Consequently:

> 'the mean partnership size of practices in 1952 was one to two GPs and in 1990 was four to five GPs. The number of practice units has consequently been reduced from almost 11 000 in 1980 to 9000 in 1990. Although only 10% of GPs are single-handed, they make up over 3000 GP units. A typical GP unit is now responsible for 8000–10 000 patients, whilst the larger practices have lists of over 20 000 patients[32].'

Staffing general-practice-based primary care

Some GPs claim that they cannot delegate, either clinically or managerially, because their staff are not up to the tasks that they would want to delegate. The workshops were not designed to provide objective evidence whether this is so, but if it is then why do not GPs demand training for those staff who are willing to develop their competence, and engage in disciplinary action with those who are not? Some examples quoted in the workshops would trigger this in other settings, but failed to do so in general practice.

There are several reasons for this, not least the fact that in many rural areas staff are also patients of the practice, thus presenting the GP as manager with a task that is unpalatable to him as the person's personal doctor. GPs, particularly in small community practices, have for so long engaged in relationships with their staff that are more 'familial' than 'managerial', that now, when someone's performance falls short of what the practice so direly needs, the GP feels unable to tackle that person managerially. Inevitably, however, these GPs and other members of staff pay an enormous price for such deadlock, not least in their own levels of stress.

If GPs and practice managers in the workshops are right in their future predictions and the government through the new health authorities begins seriously to question value for money in primary care and to look systematically at activity, outputs and outcomes in relation to inputs, this failure to tackle long-standing staffing issues will be questioned. Similarly, if practices, especially small ones, begin to 'cluster' for various reasons and particularly if two or more small practices join to fund a competent manager, this will bring pressure for change.

Recently, FHSAs have increasingly developed and applied formulae to govern practice staffing allocations and have then left practices to choose how they spend their money within their allocation. This too, in contrast with the automatic reimbursement of up to two staff per doctor which formerly applied, will push practices themselves to ensure that they are getting value for money from their existing staffing pattern and existing staff members.

Increasing external pressures on practices for greater accountability for performance will be translated into similar pressures within the practice, formalizing relationships between GPs, practice managers and staff in ways that many GPs would still consider foreign to the ethos of a small, supposedly caring organization. Formalizing relationships need not mean that they become less close, warm or personal; it does mean that the performance requirement that lies at the heart of the relationship is clarified.

Effective staff recruitment has never been a strong suit in general practice, but GPs can no longer afford to continue the often haphazard practices of yesteryear. Practice managers now take a major role in the appointment of reception and clerical staff, but these appointments are only as effective as the practice manager's own recruitment skills. Many of them, in listing their own future needs, specified personnel skills. These will be particularly important if, as many GPs and practice managers believe, they will be responsible for recruiting and managing other health professionals in the future.

Issues of staff performance, discipline and possible termination of contract are immensely painful for most practices, especially those which are small and deeply embedded in their local communities. To be forced to tackle them appears for some practices to be a baptism of fire from which a more effectively managed organization is born. One practice which made a member of staff redundant changed its whole philosophy. The difficulties they experienced throughout this process led the partners and the manager to commit themselves to recruiting better qualified and more motivated people in future.

Some practice managers experience real difficulty in introducing clear performance requirements for staff in the practice, particularly when failure to meet these results in disciplinary procedure. The GPs' support of the manager may then be tested, as staff go behind the manager's back to the GPs.

As performance management enters general practice as it has done the rest of the NHS, these challenges will be more sharply felt in these small organizations that have been run for so long on familial rather than formal organizational lines. As the next chapter shows, GPs and practice managers are aware of the inevitability of these developments and of their own needs to develop the competence and confidence to meet them.

Futures 5

Introduction

In contrast to the varied pictures of the current management function and its distribution that were presented by GPs and practice managers from different-sized practices, the futures they described were remarkably similar, although changes to practice organization and management featured more largely in the responses of the larger and fundholding practices.

Participants fully expect to have to manage in a context of continuing uncertainty which will demand of them far greater flexibility than ever before. They were convinced, however, that the future would contain the following features:

- continued and increasing demands from patients due to rising expectations of medicine and lower tolerance of pain, disability and discomfort

- continued and increasing demands from government and health commissions, with continued emphasis on 'themes' or targets

- resources becoming tighter and their allocation increasingly conditional upon production of health plans or other health authority requirements

- increased managerial responsibility for resources and increased accountability for resource use

- increased demand for evidence of organizational and clinical quality, e.g. audit (clinical and organizational), accreditation, application of clinical guidelines

- increased range of services being offered from within the practice, with implications for premises and space utilization, and for management and motivation of a wider range of individuals and groups

- increased role for practices in the clinical education of all members of the primary care team

- increased involvement beyond the practice boundary:

  i   movement of clinical activity into and out of the practice

  ii increased and closer relationships with other organizations – other practices, providers, health commissions, social services, voluntary organizations, etc.

The impact of these features will be higher workloads, longer hours and attempts by the profession and by practices to set limits, perhaps through revised, probably localized contracts which define core and non-core work.

Frequent reference was made to further development of a two-tier service and the possibility of this leading to privatization. Anxiety was also expressed about the probable increase in defensive medicine, as more clinical activity is retained within practice-based primary care. GPs recognize that this is possible only if they engage in greater delegation of clinical activity within the practice, but that this will take place against a background of increasing willingness of patients to complain. Consequently, GPs are becoming more anxious about clinical risk and and more aware of medico-legal issues.

Future careers for general practitioners and practice managers

Throughout their discussion of potential futures, GPs and practice managers referred explicitly or implicitly to potential changes in both GP and practice manager roles and careers. These changes will be influenced not simply by practice organization, but by professional organizations such as AMGP (Association of Managers in General Practice), the IHSM (Institute of Health Service Managers), the BMA (British Medical Association) and the RCGP (Royal College of General Practitioners).

The range of opportunities opening up for GPs as managers is outlined below.

Potential managerial career – GP

- *GP as doctor/director:* role adopted by GPs who wish to concentrate on clinical work within the practice; needs awareness of need for effective management in the practice; skills with small group (listening, communicating, negotiating, decision taking) to enhance functioning of partnership

- *GP with part-management portfolio:* requires understanding and competence to direct/manage that portfolio (information technology – IT, staffing, finance, etc.); capacity to work effectively with practice manager and with other partners; fostering leadership in self and others

- *Managing or executive partner:* requires modern management awareness and competence; capacity to manage professionals and the clinical–managerial interface; capacity to promote creativity within the executive partner–practice manager pair, and to manage the relationship between the pair and the rest of the organization *continued*

- *Managing beyond the practice:*

  GP education: GP tutor; course organizer; associate regional adviser; regional adviser; local faculty roles, RCGP

  Medical politics: Local Medical Committee (LMC), General Medical Services Committee (GMSC)

  NHS management as board member: trusts, commissions

  NHS management as employee: senior management roles in trusts and health authorities, including any future primary care organizations

  Inter-practice organization: consortia chief executive/clinical director/chairperson employed by the consortia or multifund

  Inter-practice–health authority: facilitator funded by the health authority to develop an emerging inter-practice organization; chair/member of various forms of GP purchasing groups

GPs are currently moving into new managerial roles with inadequate managerial preparation. With appropriate management development they could contribute much more effectively. More work needs to be done to identify more fully the management development needs of GPs moving into these roles and the most effective ways in which these could be addressed, preferably by leaders in the new health authorities, the postgraduate education system and potential providers of management development. Executive Letter EL(95)27 *Education and training in the new NHS* proposes a more collaborative approach involving purchasers, NHS health care providers, GPs and non-NHS health care providers[33].

The NHS changes of the past four years have also created considerable career opportunities for those practice managers who wish to take them. This range of opportunities is outlined below.

Potential managerial career – practice manager

- *Practice administrator*

- *Practice manager (1):* does not include practice nurse in staff accountable to practice manager; nor GPs

- *Practice manager (2):* includes practice nurse in staff organizationally accountable to practice manager, but usually not the GPs

- *Practice manager (3):* often re-titled business manager/practice developments manager/general manager: all clinical staff, including GPs and attached staff are organizationally accountable to practice manager

- *Multi-practice manager:* employed by two practices or more

- *Consortia chief executive:* usually of a fundholding consortia

- *Practice management consultant:* employed by IT or financial consultants or drug companies; independent practice, alone or in association

- *Practice management educator:* employed by university/college, or contracted in from independent base; often combined with consultancy

- *Practice/primary care development manager/facilitator:* employed by health commissions

- *Primary care commissioning/performance management:* employed by commissions

- *Chief executive, potential future primary care organizations*

Fundholding in particular spawned new roles, IT and fund management consultancy, and more lately in the management of consortia or multifunds.

A firm of recruitment consultants recently published an advertisement in the *Health Service Journal* for a chief executive of a fundholding consortia of 11 fundholding units covering a total of 28 practices[34]. The salary was quoted as 'attractive and negotiable' and the advertisement opened with the question:

> 'are you interested in making a real difference in primary care? If so, this post will provide an excellent career opportunity allowing you to play a key role in the leading edge of primary care delivery.'

The use of the term 'primary care' rather than 'general practice' is significant. The person specification includes:

> '... solid general management capability, impeccable interpersonal skills, an accomplished change manager and full appreciation of the strategic agenda, particularly GP fundholding and the internal market.'

Posts as general managers or chief executives of practice consortia and multifunds are proliferating. These posts offer an opportunity for practice managers to extend their career horizons. Their novelty and scope has already attracted managers from other parts of the NHS, a trend which will increase as the merger of FHSAs and District Health Authorities (DHAs) reduces the number of opportunities for advancement in the new health authorities. It remains to be seen whether practice managers will be attracted to working at this different level, beyond the individual practice and between several practices and the new health authority.

Those who occupy these new roles will have different development needs from those of practice managers whose prime focus is the management and development of one practice. A key issue will be whether multi-practice managerial roles develop in relation to primary care provider development or remain confined to the purchasing component. Observation so far suggests that while multi-practice organizations and roles are stimulated initially by the need for GPs to influence purchasing of hospital and community health services, the emerging organizations, by promoting communication and networking among practices, also promote developments in primary care provision.

In the two areas of Wessex from which workshop participants were drawn there is now a small but increasing number of GPs and practice managers who are interested in the development of primary care beyond the practice[35]. The need to influence the purchasing process provided the initial spur to interpractice networking, in both fundholding and non-fundholding practices, particularly among GPs.

The workshops demonstrated that people develop their understanding, orientation and skills *through direct experience* of new areas of work, particularly when offered the opportunity to reflect on this. The new health authorities could usefully promote secondments of GPs and practice managers who are already demonstrating a capacity to build effective interpractice relationships. Many FHSAs and health commissions across the country have espoused commitment to primary care development, but have rarely staffed this effort with those who know practice-based primary care from the inside. Such experiments will not be easy. Many practices would not welcome such boundary crossing and those occupying the boundary role would need support from both organizations.

Implications for management development

Both GPs and practice managers from all practices recognized the huge management implications of the futures they had described. These are grouped under the four categories of skills, personal qualities, changes in behaviour and needs. They are presented without discussion as a check-list for providers of management education and development.

Some of the items are not as narrow as they first appear. When a GP and a small group of practice managers subsequently developed their specification for a negotiation skills workshop, they realized how germane these skills were to management generally and that effective negotiating behaviours were underpinned by concepts and insights from a range of disciplines.

Skills required

- analytical skills
- information management: information access, timeliness, exchange data collection, analysis, presentation
- health and business planning
- health needs assessment
- auditing – external and internal
- finance/resource management – budgets, control, forecasting
- public relations, marketing
- estate management
- presentation skills
- survey skills
- human resource management: recruitment, appraisal, training, discipline, motivation, termination; creating and managing 'career' structures within the practice; self-development skills
- time management and delegation
- assertiveness
- stress management, coping skills

- communication skills (GPs and practice managers tend not to include within this communication strategies)

- team building

- negotiation

- liaison skills, managing interfaces with increasing numbers of other organizations

- decision making and implementing

- managing an expanding range of services, which means managing a more complex organizational structure (inter-clinical and clinical–managerial boundaries)

- managing meetings, group skills (especially for GPs)

- managing the practice–patient(s) interface.

Personal qualities required

GPs in particular like to list the *personal qualities* they feel will be necessary in surviving the future. They tend to see managers as born rather than made, although this is gradually changing as they work alongside managers who demonstrate a distinctive capacity, perspective and approach. Whereas the following personal qualities were listed by workshop GPs, they imply competencies and behaviours which can be learned:

- self-confidence

- mutual respect (GP–GP, GP–practice manager)

- fast on one's feet

- openness, honesty

- increased GP capacity to 'hear' practice manager and staff

- ability to make things happen

- literate, including IT literate

- logical
- knows own limits
- leadership/followership
- vision/antennae
- flexibility, adaptability
- greater maturity in GPs, less of the prima donna (said by GP)
- lateral thinking
- doers, delegators
- articulate
- politically aware
- enabler, not dictator.

Changes in behaviour

GPs and practice managers identified those changes in behaviour that would be needed to meet the future with confidence. As behaviours, they link to the skills and qualities listed above. More importantly, they offer a check-list for any management development provider who seeks to offer a comprehensive practice-based primary care management programme.

Changes included the need to:

- question our basic assumptions
- build uncertainty into our plans – contingencies, instability
- build flexibility into our organizations
- monitor workloads more
- set caring limits

- develop the corporate identity of the practice
- develop the whole organizational and managerial structure
- develop the primary health care team
- clarify the responsibilities of the GP
- make the practice more 'businesslike', entrepreneurial, competitive
- become more strategic
- adopt a more proactive management style, creating time to think/review through more delegation
- make the practice more accountable
- review regularly skill mix, staff capabilities/development needs
- encourage staff involvement, initiative
- recruit more rationally/objectively; no 'passengers'; more flexible contracts
- take a more structured approach to work across the whole organization: decision–action–review
- agree what is management between the management professional and the clinical professional
- employ good practice/general manager with financial expertise and appropriate management style to manage professionals and act as catalyst
- lead by example in giving/exchanging responsibilities
- develop greater contextual understanding – political economy of health, business management, so we can learn from but also critique inappropriate applications to health care
- develop more effective interpartner relationships, acceptability of protocols

- implement as doctors the decisions agreed as directors
- to act as a team first, and as individuals second
- identify and develop leadership capacity in GPs and practice managers for roles inside and outside the practice
- develop career choices for GPs.

Needs

In due course health commissions will become the new health authorities. This list contains items GPs and practice managers said they would need from the bodies that would hold them accountable in the future:

- time to think
- better communications with health commissions, support from them in practical ways
- availability of management consultancy
- clarification from health commissions on finance/support for management education and development for GP and practice managers
- bigger staff budgets, more space, better IT that is suited to our business, customized to the practice, workflow software
- huge upgrade in IT staff – perhaps spread across several practices; health commission could contract in IT training specialist who would train interested GPs and practice managers, who would then 'cascade' the competence through other practices
- fewer hidden agendas
- period of consolidation to assess benefits of GP fundholding to the population

- GP fundholders need budgets sufficient to sustain innovation

- incentives for realizable targets

- define core content of general practice and ensure add-ons are funded in terms of both finance and manpower

- all primary care team under our management (funded) accountable to us (from larger practices group)

- fewer middle men/women in grey suits, paper shuffling

- patients taking more responsibility for their own care

- GP input to locality purchasing.

Management development needs

The GPs and practice managers recognized the management development implications of the requisite skills, personal qualities and changes in behaviour they identified. GPs in particular are becoming more aware that they need much more management development, but are also prone to say 'we don't know what it is we need to know'.

Awareness of the content of 'subjects' such as management and the political economy of health care (rather than straight health economics) would help GPs and practice managers locate themselves more clearly in the new NHS landscape, but realistically only a tiny minority of them would wish or would have the time to study these subject areas in depth. There are, however, concepts and conceptual frameworks within these subjects that could be usefully offered as part of management education and development.

Only a small minority of practice managers and an even smaller minority of GPs seek formal management education that results in a management qualification, such as a Master of Business Administration (MBA) degree or a Diploma or

Certificate in Management Studies (DMS,CMS), although numbers will probably increase in the future as career options expand. Those workshop participants who had sought formal management education had done so for a range of reasons. Some sought a qualification or formal credential for career advancement; some practice managers sought the experience of higher education because they had missed this earlier in their career and felt it would give them more confidence when relating to an increasingly graduate managerial and professional population; some expressed an emergent interest in management *per se*, beginning to see this as a subject or discipline as well as an activity.

Formal management education in a university or college was seen to offer the opportunity to study 'general management' rather than 'practice management', to learn about different types of organizations in different types of industries and sectors and to mix with managers from them. It was hoped that this broader comparative perspective would bring new insights into the management of their own organization and 'industry'. This was particularly attractive to a GP who was completing an MBA.

The development of a primary-care-led NHS would probably be furthered by encouraging and offering some financial support to the relatively small number of GPs and practice managers who wish to undertake broader-based management education programmes. Financial support could be made conditional upon project work and dissertation being focused on areas agreed by the student and the funders, and subsequently made available to funding organizations. Funders may also wish to require that, if successful, students agree to act as mentors to other GPs or practice managers who may wish to undertake formal management education.

Concerns have been expressed that formal management education is too theoretical and insufficiently linked to the needs of learners in their organizational roles and to the needs of those organizations who may be financially supporting the learning. Business schools have become more aware of these concerns in recent years, and now tend to ensure that their programmes are linked more closely to the needs of learners and their sponsoring organizations.

Quite the contrary concern could be expressed about much of what has been done in the name of management development for GPs and practice managers, which has been largely skills-based. There is nothing wrong with this, and indeed GPs, but more particularly practice managers, have repeatedly asked for opportunities to develop and enhance particular skills. The risk is that while discrete skills may be enhanced, learners have often not been helped to locate these in a broader framework of managerial understanding. The effect has been to focus practice management constantly at the operational level.

The capacity of practices to manage their own future depends on the skill with which they create and sustain their organization's capacity for both reactive and pre-emptive change. Capacity is defined as:

> 'to take in or hold . . . ability to take in impressions, ideas, knowledge . . . mental receiving power . . . the active power of mind . . . capability, possibility.'[36]

High capacity individuals are more to able take in and to process environmental impressions.

Organizations which wish to survive and thrive must develop this same capacity to scan, take in and process signals from the environment.

Whatever management development programmes or activities are offered in the future for GPs and practice managers, they must include means of helping them develop a fast and flexible organizational 'intelligence' function in their own practices, which will promote their own and their practice's capacity to learn and adapt.

Formative management development experience | 6

Introduction

GPs and practice managers attending the workshops were asked to describe experiences and events that had contributed to their development as managers. They were encouraged to include life experience, previous work experience and not just formal training. Subsequently, formative participants wished to see some of these experiences included in formal training programmes, for example the opportunity to learn from observing other practices and from sharing problems and issues with others doing the same job, and with other managers in different kinds of organizations, including the NHS and business and commerce.

GPs and practice managers are pragmatic in their approach to management learning. The majority have learned by doing. In the early 1980s the only management courses being offered were very short events for GPs at the King's Fund College and subsequently for GPs and practice managers at the Royal College of General Practitioners. The Association of Health Centre and Practice Administrators (AHCPA) and the Association of Medical Secretaries and Receptionists (AMSPAR) both developed diplomas, and the Vocational Training Scheme in

General Practice began to offer a management component within its curriculum.

In the early 1990s, with the introduction of the 1990 Contract, fundholding and other NHS changes, educational institutions, freelance consultants, drug companies, publishers and FHSAs began to engage in practice management development. Much of this activity also comprises one- or two-day courses that are skills-based with titles such as business planning, time management, personnel and negotiating skills.

Participants' experience of these activities will be presented later in this chapter. The next three sections focus on other experiences which were felt to have contributed to these GPs' and practice managers' development as managers.

'Sitting next to Nellie'

Several GPs and practice managers initially became interested in management from observing others. One GP's father ran a restaurant, enabling the GP when quite young to develop 'a feel for business' and for recognizing the skills of others.

These observed others became either positive or negative role models. One GP who is a school governor observed an effective chairman, watched him create a management process in which he identified people's expertise and used it appropriately in small task groups. He learned something from this that was vital to the management of general practice, namely that while governors might not get on as individuals, they functioned as a group because they were well-managed and trained. He also observed that this chairman took care to construct a physical and social setting appropriate to the work.

A practice manager from the city offices of one of the big clearing banks valued a manager there who was perceived to be calm, well organized and assertive. He always had the facts and in meetings was often quiet, sitting back and listening. His

desk was always clear and he protected himself from involvement in day-to-day issues. Another practice manager's role
model had trusted staff and demonstrated this, knew the staff
and their individual expertise well, and had previously done
the job herself. Another practice manager had worked with a
practice manager who saw herself on a level with the GPs, had
developed staff, encouraged training and was forward-think-
ing 14 years ago. Another learned from a woman manager in
a firm who was 'in control, friendly, self-confident and a huge
success'. This practice manager also learned while at this firm
to work with a very demanding person, recognizing that this
'felt OK because you felt valued'. Another manager learned a
great deal from her husband who is a manager.

Role models can be negative as well as positive: observing
his single-handed GP father convince one GP participant that
he would never want to work in that way.

Previous work experience

Many previous work experiences were formative for both GPs
and managers: running a company; running a family; running
a haulage contracting firm in which a practice manager had
learned to manage diverse people. The lorry drivers were
highly individualistic – very like GPs. Another practice
manager who had been a teacher, then a head teacher, found
that her skills were transferable to the practice, particularly in
working with both doctors and patients. She had learned to
work to individuals' strengths.

Several GPs and practice managers spoke of being given
responsibility slightly beyond that which they felt capable of at
the time. Some individuals referred to 'being thrown in at the
deep end and having to do management', whereas others
referred to being given responsibility but with sufficient support.

One GP found himself challenged by the transition from trainee to principal, and several GPs valued the young principals' groups which had helped them through this transition.

Some practice managers contrasted the environment in commerce and its emphasis on the importance of training with that in general practice which faced so many challenges with little systematic preparation for them. The contrast was also observed by GPs and practice managers with a background in the armed services where they had received structured training and experience. In the services they had observed a clearly defined management structure, the importance of delegation and of leadership – all of which seemed foreign to the culture of general practice.

This same theme of development through change was mentioned by several GPs and practice managers who referred to living through crises and huge changes in their organizations, particularly in the past few years. The next section will indicate the importance of opportunities to share and talk through this experience in order to learn from it. Some GP–practice manager pairs, particularly those who had led their practices into fundholding, said that they had learned a lot from going through this process together.

Comparative observation and experience

Of greatest value to both GPs and practice managers was the opportunity to compare oneself and one's organization with others. In part, this reflects the isolation of practices until very recently, and there is no doubt that practice managers have led the way in reducing this.

Several younger GPs referred to the valuable experience they had gained from their training practices and from doing locum work. Both experiences enabled them to select aspects of management and organization they valued and would try to apply to their own practice, and to identify aspects that were better avoided. One GP argued that young GPs should be able to move around before settling into partnership, an opportunity recommended in two recent papers on postgraduate education in general practice[37, 38]. Despite the value so many GPs and practice managers place upon comparative experience, few GPs move and most GPs continue to take a dim view of those who do so.

Few practice managers move although there are indications of a greater willingness to do so in the future. Practice managers gain comparative experience at second hand through their membership of local practice manager groups established by the FHSA/health commission, the Association of Managers in General Practice (AMGP) or themselves. Practice managers are even more isolated in their practices than GPs, because most of them are still in the position of a minority of one. They need to share their thinking, and feeling, with others doing the same job in a rapidly changing occupation. One of the practice managers at the workshops had jointly established a small support group for practice managers, the members of which bought in their own facilitator.

More recently, fundholding spawned much more inter-practice communication with the formation of fundholder groups and locality groups of non-fundholders. Some GPs and practice managers valued the opportunities these offered for learning from other practices' experience in addressing particular issues.

Several GPs and practice managers also referred to the learning they had gained from having a management consultant in the practice. The contribution of consultants stems in part from their comparative experience of organizations against which a practice's organizational understanding and behaviour can be 'tested'. Some GPs and practice managers said that the organization development consultancy attached to writing their health plan had offered an opportunity for self as well as organizational review.

Most GPs and practice managers had to learn by doing, but this was difficult without structured opportunities to reflect on that doing and to obtain feedback from others. These were the opportunities that were sought from future training programmes.

Formative training experiences – general practitioners

Most GPs' accounts of training experiences that had helped them become managerially more effective omitted any reference to postgraduate medical education. Only one GP, probably the youngest of the GP participants, recalled receiving any management education in the Vocational Training Scheme (VTS) or finding the VTS helpful. A few GPs had found working in the training practice helpful, but seem not to have been offered any structured opportunities to reflect on their organizational observation there.

It may be that despite the best efforts of those GP educators in charge of the VTS, the GPs in training are oriented towards becoming clinically rather than managerially competent in general practice so that they do not absorb what is offered by way of management education. It is also probable that most of the GPs who attended these workshops trained 10 or more years ago when the VTS contained little if anything on 'management' beyond knowledge of the Red Book's terms and conditions of service (*The Statement of Fees and Allowances Payable to General Medical Practitioners in England and Wales*; prepared under Regulation 24).

Many, particularly the younger ones, were critical of basic medical education for containing nothing on management. One GP argued that 'you must get business skills and accounting into basic medical education'. It is notoriously difficult to introduce new areas of learning into the medical curriculum, but a strategic shift from secondary to primary care and the development of a primary-care-led NHS will elude the government and the NHS Executive unless radical changes are made rapidly to medical education, at both undergraduate and postgraduate levels.

A review of management education for general practice is urgently needed. Ideally, this would see basic medical education, the VTS and continuing medical education as a coherent whole for management education and development purposes. While many GPs may not wish to become managers themselves, even in their own practices, they are employers in those practices and will consequently influence if not determine the quality of practice management therein. They will also increasingly be expected to influence the direction of policy and management in the NHS.

While participating in the VTS as a student was not seen as helpful in developing managerial capacity, some GPs found that being a trainer within the Scheme promoted their own learning, as trainers were offered opportunities to observe others' practices, to reflect on comparisons and to share learning with others. Being a trainer also offered access to further training courses such as one on group dynamics, which one GP trainer found could be useful to his own organization.

Some GPs had found the local Royal College Faculty Annual Course useful, particularly as it contained visits to other practices, but other GPs had not even heard of this course. Positive reference was also made to workshops run by particularly gifted educators; to a speed reading course; and to having a management student from a local business school on placement in the practice.

Two GPs were school governors and praised the training programme they had received. They saw a video on teacher selection and had gone through a simulated selection process. One GP had taken the video back to the practice and shown it to staff.

Another GP had been greatly stimulated by participating in a part-time MBA programme at his local university. He had learned a great deal from working with managers outside the NHS; from having to think and write about his 'industry' (health care) nationally and internationally; and from learning, from a manager of an international bank, how to 'get at the business through the numbers'. Management consultants had, with very few exceptions, been found valuable in developing GPs' own management learning and that of the practice as a whole.

GPs also valued the residential Primary Care Team Development workshops sponsored locally by the FHSA, but acknowledged difficulties in transferring learning back into the practice as a whole.

One GP valued a distance learning package on time management because he had been able to do it in his own time and at his own pace, and it required him to fill in time sheets on which he received feedback. This had enabled him to modify his own behaviour.

Other GPs referred to the value of young principals' groups, trainers' groups, Balint groups, and RCGP-based groups in enabling them to develop managerially, again probably because of the inherent interpractice comparisons these made possible.

Some also referred to the John Cleese/Video Arts management films which were seen as enjoyable, informative and highly professional. Their 'lessons' were clear and easy to recall.

Formative training experiences – practice managers

The most cited training experiences for managers were those offered by AHCPA (Association of Health Centre and Practice Administrators, now AMGP – Association of Managers in General Practice). The three-day annual course, held nationally, the quarterly meetings held regionally and AHCPA's Open University (OU) initiative were all praised.

AMGP events offer the opportunity to come together with other practice managers who face the same challenges; to share observations, reflections and understanding; and to cross-fertilize ideas. They tend to be run by people in practice for people in practice, and as such they develop the competence and confidence of those managers who have been promoted from within the practice staff. This is a vital function, but as some of these managers develop an interest in management *per se*, they need something different.

AMGP's association with the OU offers practice managers the opportunity to begin to acquire formal management qualifications at their own pace, in their own place. One practice manager found the books used became a permanent source of reference, and tutorials offered the opportunity to compare experience with managers in the broader NHS and beyond. The OU course also offers telephone tutor group contact which was valued by practice managers who can feel isolated within their own organizations. One practice manager said that the OU experience had made her more open to and tolerant of others' ideas.

AMGP is moving with the times[39] and responding to the challenge it faces in containing within one organization members who are still entering practice management from the ranks of practice staff and those who are now capable of leaving practice management to become audit and organization development consultants to practices.

As practice management expanded as an occupation and people came in from outside practices, the IHSM (Institute of Health Services Management) registered its interest by holding for the first time a national practice managers' conference and exhibition in Birmingham in 1993 – this is now a yearly event. Some managers had been stimulated by this, again because of the opportunity to share experience and learn from that of others across the country.

One-day skills courses offered by FHSAs/health commissions often met a particular need at a particular point in time, or because they were offered in response to requests from them. These courses need to be located into a coherent strategy of management development based on individual, practice and health authority needs. The development of such a strategy should become more feasible as a result of the establishment of local consortia of the various stakeholders in practice-based primary care development[33]. The development of a modified internal market in primary care education may loosen some of the rigidities that have formerly perpetuated the separate development of the various primary care professions.

Managers found some difficulty in consolidating and reflecting on their learning because of the amount of work waiting at the practice the following day. These courses tend to be fitted into a busy week and do not engage the self of the manager in the same way as longer courses, regularly held learning groups or events such as the AMGP annual course or the IHSM conference. Practice managers welcomed the opportunity offered by the national, annual events to think about the development of practice management as an occupation and by implication the development of their occupational identity.

Because of the newness of the occupation, the professional isolation of managers in their own practice situations and the challenge of managing in organizations owned by those who also work at the coalface, practice managers' use of self in the managerial role is central to their effectiveness. One female practice manager had previously been trained in counselling, which had enhanced her self-confidence and enabled her to use her self quite consciously in the managerial role.

Several female managers from outside bring with them experience of general management courses which they find valuable in coming to terms with the practice as an organization. Managers who have grown from within the practice differ in their evaluation of general management programmes, such as the Diploma in Management Studies (DMS). For some, the experience broadens their horizons, giving them a more objective view of their own organizational setting and themselves within it, while for others 'it just does not impinge on what I do'.

Whether such a negative comment reflects on the quality of the course, in particular its lack of relevance to partnership organizations, or on the orientations and aspirations of the manager is not clear. Managers in the workshops tended to fall into two major groups: those who saw themselves in a job entitled 'practice manager' which it was unlikely they would ever leave, and then only to do a similar job; and those who saw themselves as part of the rapidly developing occupation and career of practice management which might lead not only to more challenging posts in general practice, but to as yet undelineated managerial posts in primary care development, the broader NHS or even outside.

In pursuing their own management development, those in this latter group will seek general management courses, not necessarily because they aspire to move beyond practice management, but because they are often in practices which are transforming themselves as primary care providers and as purchasers of secondary care. Although these are not primary care *businesses* in the sense of being private companies, they are nevertheless organized on increasingly businesslike lines. These managers know that some version of the internal market will probably enter primary care and that primary care versions of performance indicators, value for money and efficiency indices are not far off. They, and their like-minded GPs, want to be able to take the initiative and not be confined always to reacting to government and local health authority policies.

They are still a relatively small group, but as health authorities increasingly attempt to influence the recruitment and development of practice managers, they will grow in number and their management development needs are very different from those of the first group.

Management development needs

7

Introduction

GPs' and practice managers' recollections of the experiences they felt had made them better managers were often drawn from their own work experience: through observing people they deemed to be effective managers; through 'being dropped in at the deep end'; through visiting or working in similar, or different, organizations to their own; to having the opportunity to discuss their work with others in the same field.

Many found the workshops a rich learning experience, in that they offered an opportunity to reflect on the experience of recent years, to work through feelings about the NHS changes and begin to develop an understanding of their origins and broader context. Many participants expressed concern about GPs and practice managers who had not had the opportunity to attend or who did not avail themselves of it.

Their concerns imply that as a general rule future management development activities should always attempt to offer opportunities to enhance understanding and to work through feelings, as well as to develop and enhance skills.

The first requirement of any management development strategy for practice-based primary care is that it take account of the acute variation in need for management development in the wide range of GPs and practice managers who attended these workshops. Levels of managerial and organizational awareness, interest, experience and expertise vary enormously. Unless this is taken into account, money and time will be wasted, and GPs and practice managers will be demotivated rather than motivated by management development.

Management development specifications by general practitioners and practice managers

Workshop participants were asked to work up in groups, specifications for desired management development or education experiences. They found this a difficult exercise as it required them to think through something that would meet a need they considered important, whereas they themselves were intent on using the occasion of the workshops to work on their own needs there and then. This meant that if they chose to design an event which aimed to develop the capacity to organize interpractice local groupings, much of the discussion was spent on sharing their experience of trying to do this locally.

The subjects of their specifications are listed below and some examples are given in Appendix II.

Focus of management education and development specifications

- Developing a forum for sharing information

- A structured approach to the development of practice managers/practice management

continued

- Organizing interpractice local groupings/an inter-practice organization (2)

- Comprehensive management programme for GPs

- Negotiation skills workshop

- A framework for management development for practice managers

- Management of change (2)

- Developing people skills

- Managing time

- Decision management (2)

- Primary health care team development

- Organization and management development plan for three practices sharing some facilities on a new joint site

- Developing performance indicators in general practice

- Programme to learn more about locality groups

- Workshop for GPs: using your practice manager effectively

- Structured practice visiting as a learning device

- Assertiveness training

- Integrated management development/What would an integrated programme look like?(2)

- NVQ and practice management

More important than the detailed content of the specifications is what they convey about the priorities and preoccupations of participants and their preferred approaches to learning. Key themes are outlined as follows.

Integrating individual management development and practice organization development

Some GPs and practice managers had been excited by former training experiences but had then been frustrated by their difficulties in implementing their learning back in the practice. Consequently, they were concerned to effect more integration of individual management development and practice organization development.

This is a challenging issue for the new health authorities. Organization development (OD) is expensive, but it addresses the needs of the whole practice. One of the OD consultants who worked with some of the practices represented on the workshops suggested that it was difficult to do OD with practices whose GPs and managers were minimally aware of management, as both an issue within their organizations and as a discipline.

If health authorities are to invest in the management education and development of individual GPs and practice managers, they will need to assure themselves that providers of that education and development do all they can to ensure that the learner is able to apply their learning to the development of their organization. This can be ensured by making their own organizations the focus of at least some assignments and presentations.

One advantage of management education and development over organization development is that individuals are given structured opportunities 'to think the unthinkable' with others from *outside* their own organizations or industries. A small number of GPs and practice managers in the workshops are already envisioning a new primary care system whose organizations have yet to come into being. It is precisely because general practices have for so long been insular that general management development for some GPs and practice managers is now so crucial.

Promoting interpractice organization development through management development

The need to develop more effective interpractice relationships emerged repeatedly in the workshops, a sign that GPs in particular are beginning to recognize interpractice structures and processes as a major feature of their future landscape. While the development of locality groups was chosen as the focus, this is only one variant of *interorganizational relationships* which were a major feature of the 'futures' described by participants, including relationships with the health authorities, trusts, social services, the voluntary sector and self-help groups.

Few GPs and practice managers enjoy access to the emerging literature on *interorganizational and intersectoral collaboration,* yet many of them are aware of literature and professional development opportunities which focus on *interprofessional collaboration.* These two types of literature tend to progress along different channels but creative linkages could be made by small learning groups of GPs and practice managers who were offered an opportunity to use the literature to work on their own local and practice issues. This particular example also suggests a need to involve more aware GPs and practice managers in research and development (R&D) in primary care. If a primary-care-led NHS is to become a reality, primary care will need to secure a greater proportion of R&D funds. Professors and regional advisers in general practice will champion such a shift in funding and the involvement of greater numbers of GPs in research, but if the organizational as well as the clinical capacity of practice-based primary care is to be developed, then greater involvement of practice managers in research and development would be a productive use of funds.

An integrated comprehensive approach to management development

Several specifications designed by workshop participants required them to think through a 'structured', 'integrated' or 'comprehensive' approach to management development for practice managers and/or GPs. These arose from the emerging preoccupation in several of the workshops with the need for:

- *a diagnostic approach* to individual management development needs and a programme that would be grounded in these

- a programme that would offer *opportunity to broaden contextual understanding* of both health care policy and modern management, as well as offering to enhance skills.

Diagnostic service

> 'Most of us are still at the diagnostic end. We have not even defined properly what we need. We can say what our wants are but the needs are different.' (practice manager)

GPs in particular often confessed that 'we don't know what it is that we need to know', and emphasized their need for a management development diagnostic facility or service. New career opportunities are emerging for GPs and practice managers both inside and outside the practice. Some are more sharply aware of this than others, but over the next few years increasing numbers of GPs and practice managers will need help in deciding what kind of managerial career they want and the management development they will need in order to pursue it.

General practitioners

Having developed an interest in management, some GPs experience the dilemma of 'shall I be clinician or manager, or both, and in what proportions?' and would welcome an opportunity to work through this dilemma with someone who has the time and the competence to help. They are dismissive of their existing careers guidance arrangement, arguing that this is staffed by 'oldies out to grass'. Retired GPs have no experience of the kind of environment in which mid-life and younger GPs now practise.

Almost all GPs criticized their medical and even their GP training for its failure to prepare them for management, and although they acknowledged that many of the skills they learned in becoming GPs were relevant to management, few made the connection or saw it as legitimate. They also felt that these were people skills and that what they lacked was an understanding of modern management and of the national and international health care context in which they were working.

Some GPs are becoming so interested in management as a discipline that they are seeking management education or development themselves. If this involves any more than simple skills workshops then it will always be potentially destabilizing, firstly for the GP and secondly for the practice. The experience will probably affect the GP's own identity and potentially change the relative balance of clinician and manager within that identity. Consequently, it may shift the current distribution of the management function within the practice.

In the workshops every position on this spectrum of identity was represented, from GPs who really wanted to be clinicians but felt they could only protect their right to do this by totally controlling their organization through to a GP who was thinking of giving up clinical work to become a manager. Some partnerships have now agreed to give a particular partner the equivalent of clinical sessions in which to exercise a management role within the practice, although this is more typical of fundholding practices. In one of the counties from which participants were drawn, one GP is seconded two days a week as general manager of a new primary care organization. Another is financed to service and co-ordinate a locality group of non-fundholding GPs.

GPs as independent contractors in their own organizations find it more difficult to pursue a paid managerial role, whether inside or outside the practice. There is a big issue for the NHS here. If the government is genuinely committed to producing a primary-care-led NHS, it will need more GPs to make a management contribution not only within their practices but outside. Millions of pounds have been invested in management development for consultants, particularly those who were to become clinical directors, together with considerable investment in management education for senior registrars. In comparison, little has gone into management development for GPs.

This investment is now vital, not least so that GPs learn what *not* to manage and what they can safely delegate, providing they make effective practice manager appointments, so that they spend their intelligence, time and energy on what they, preferably, *must* manage.

If GPs themselves do not understand management adequately, they will not delegate sufficiently. They will continue to feel ambivalent about practice management and possibly also their practice manager. Good GP–practice manager relationships depend on GPs' acknowledgement of the need for an effectively managed practice and on their understanding of the prerequisites of effective management.

GPs in these workshops, even those from the larger practices, commented that doctors find functioning in groups very difficult, particularly if they have to take decisions. Some said that even in group practice they did not work clinically as a group and that to work in a group 'you have to give something'. What they have to give is the willingness to follow when one of their colleagues leads. For GPs this is chronically difficult.

Practice managers

Practice managers also vary greatly in their management development needs, depending upon the work they currently do, their level of aspiration and particularly whether they want a job or a career. Overall, women practice managers tend not to be as assertive as men, although there are striking exceptions to this generalization. The generalization applies, however, not simply to their interactions with GPs in the course of their work, but in their own diagnosis of their development needs and their pursuit of means of meeting those needs.

Those who are most clear about their needs are those managers, mainly women, who have *grown from within* their practices and want to go on growing. They tend, like some of the enthusiastic GPs, to want to gain a broader and deeper understanding of modern management and of health care policy development.

Some are currently considering their own development needs and speak of embarking on courses that would yield a qualification such as an MBA (Master of Business Administration) or the DMS (Diploma in Management Studies). When asked to identify what they thought these educational experiences would offer, these managers spoke of being helped to articulate their own vision for the organizations in which they worked. They also spoke of now having to relate to far more senior levels of people outside their own organizations, a development of the past two years which they expected to continue and intensify in the future. The 'time out' offered by such management development programmes was perceived also to offer 'time with' people not only from other practices, but from a broader range of organizations.

These women managers had grown from within the practices which employed them and been encouraged by their GPs to extend their range of work and to push the boundaries of their competence. These women, and others in the workshops, appeared to need a certain level of *confidence* before they could go out and get the level of *competence* they now so obviously seek.

Those practice managers who now seek to manage larger, more complex practice-based primary care organizations would gain from the assessment centre and mentoring activity that has been made available in the NHS General Management Training Scheme and some of the Opportunity 2000 programmes sponsored by the Women's Unit of the NHS Executive.

Little career guidance is available within the practice, because the practice manager is professionally in a minority of one. Sympathetic GPs may supply a sounding board and encouragement, but they are not usually aware of the range of management development activities that might be available, nor have they the skills to help the manager choose appropriately.

This service could be supplied by the new health authorities' personnel departments, but the evidence from our workshops suggests that practice managers could be loath to air their self-doubts and anxieties to those who are increasingly playing a role in their appointment, pay and conditions; neither would GPs welcome this.

The new health authorities could enter into consultancy arrangements with firms or university and college departments who might offer such a service, but confidentiality of consultation should be assured. This is in no way to discount the training and development activities offered by former FHSAs and health commissions, nor the organization and team development activities they funded. These activities often supported practice managers in their views of what was necessary in practices and helped them more effectively to put those views into practice.

The need for a diagnostic service is particularly acute for practice managers. In part, this relates to widespread lack of appraisal of practice managers by GPs. Even where this exists, both GPs and practice managers recognize its limitations because of the GP's own lack of management development. It is an appraisal by an employer rather than a manager. There are also obvious limitations to its effectiveness with senior and highly experienced practice managers who may be ready to move beyond the single practice focus. GPs, understandably, have neither career counselling skills nor in most cases sufficient awareness of potential future developments to be able to offer the kind of service practice managers are seeking.

Mentoring

Programmes for women managers in the NHS sponsored by the Women's Unit of the NHS Executive already promote mentoring, one of the fastest growing management development activities. The activity is even more vital to the development of women managers in singular management positions located in organizations which are owned and controlled by non-managers in the professional sense of the term.

Jenny Sweeney, Senior Consultant at the Industrial Society, argues that 'progression (for women managers) depends on being able to manage the power in an organization . . . (and that) . . . you can't be trained to do that. You have to learn it through talking to others who've done it, by example and role model', which is what many practice managers were saying in the workshops.

An increasing cadre of practice managers are capable of mentoring colleagues and probably do so on an informal basis. A development programme could be offered to established practice managers who would like to mentor others. This could begin with a two-day residential programme in which participants:

- identified the aims and prerequisites of effective mentoring

- identified their own positive and negative experiences of being mentored, and what could be learned from them

- identified the ethics of mentoring and means of ensuring these were observed

- practised mentoring with the help of video techniques.

This group could come together in a consultation or supervision group on a regular basis for further learning based on their own mentoring commitments. It would be in the interests of health authorities to finance an experimental programme and to pay those who had successfully completed it as formally accredited practice manager mentors within their area. A minimum structure of accountability would need to be established which observed the confidentiality of the mentoring relationship.

Gains to health authorities from mentors continuing to meet in a group would be the opportunity to abstract from their shared experience those issues that emerged in most of their mentoring assignments, which might then be addressed in other arenas such as formal courses or workshops for practice managers and GPs.

The alternative is to offer an externally based mentor, who could be university or consultancy based, or to encourage existing women practice managers in particular to use managers in the rest of the NHS or in business. The risk is that these would have an inadequate grasp of the nature of general practice organizations, although sometimes this can be helpfully challenging to practice managers who have known nothing else.

Those practice managers who have entered practice management from established careers outside could also be encouraged to become mentors. They might also wish to seek a mentor for a time in the course of their transition into practice management. It should not be assumed that they have no mentoring needs. There is always a risk that these practice managers are seen as the 'real' or 'professional' managers, with the assumption that their management development needs were met long ago in their previous organizations.

Health authorities must beware colluding with such assumptions. It is not in the interests of practice-based primary care development for there to develop a 'them-and-us', outsiders/insiders culture of practice management. This does not mean that the differences between the two groups should be denied; rather than they should be identified as potential resources which each group can offer the other. Health authorities need to encourage the involvement of all practice managers in local practice manager liaison groups.

Presentation skills development for female practice managers

From so many of the small groups of practice managers within the workshops, the men reported back in the large group. From the mixed groups, typically a GP would report back, but on occasions a male practice manager. Many women practice managers admitted that presenting material publicly, even in a small group, provoked great anxiety and that 'it never got easier'.

High quality, sensitively run presentation skills programmes would result not only in increased competence but more importantly in increased confidence on the part of women practice managers. A number of quite visionary female practice managers were still hesitant to express their vision within the practice.

All management development activity for women practice managers should require and support maximum participation in their own learning. Facilitated learning groups in which one focus is the manager's use of self in the group as an analogue of her use of self in the practice would promote this development.

The partnership, the practice manager and practice management

GPs and practice managers need help in thinking through their relationship and the nature of their organization. Organizations that formed the basis of traditional management theory were pyramidal in shape and hierarchical in nature, and contained an assumption that responsibility, accountability – and often capacity – increased from the bottom to the top.

Management's 'model of man' and of human motivation has always been antipathetic to most professionals who apply to their work a model of organization that is a mix of colleague-ship and independence. Professionalism and managerialism are in themselves belief systems about the best way of organizing work[11,12].

The antipathy of many if not most doctors towards 'management' might usefully be reinterpreted as an antipathy to 'managerialism' as ideology. Similarly, the attitudes of many NHS managers towards doctors is one of challenge to and rejection of 'professionalism' as a means of organizing work. The languages of the two belief systems are very different: whereas managers speak of accountability, doctors speak of responsibility.

Modern management thinking is taking on board the complexity of the contemporary and probable future organization of work that is increasingly going to be done by 'professional' people working together in teams. Much of the emerging literature is remarkably relevant to the management of practice-based primary care, but *very* few GPs and practice managers have access to it.

They increasingly have access to management consultancy and through this some have adopted the model of the partnership as a board of directors, with an executive partner if any as chairman of the board, the practice manager as manager and the GPs in doctor role as one group of the several staff groups within the practice.

The distinctions offered by the model, between doctor as director and doctor as manager, and between directors and manager, seem to change GPs' feelings about managing and the threat of 'being managed'. It seems to reassure them that they can relinquish much of the routine management demands without losing control of the really important issues. It also allows them to see that being accountable to the practice manager organizationally when they are in doctor role is being accountable to him or her as their agent, hence to themselves. In any event, practice managers' status as employees ensures that they control anything or anyone in the practice wholly within the limits of authority delegated to them by their employers, the GPs.

What the model does not do is relieve the GPs of developing a consensus as directors. It does not alter the partnership and its dynamics; it tackles only the relationship between the doctors, when managing and when doctoring, and the practice manager. Achieving consensus within the partnership is more difficult, because it is that point in the organization at which clinical and managerial intersect *within the individual* (the GPs are *both doctors and directors*).

It is also where the organization (the practice) and the profession (general practice) intersect. When a management consultant promotes a discussion with partners about questions such as 'Who are we? What's special about us? What do we want to become?', responses frequently reveal major differences in definitions of 'good general practice' and of the appropriate balance to strike between being a business *and* a profession, or between 'practitioner' or 'practice' models of care[2]. The 1990 GP Contract and fundholding tested many partnerships to breaking point, precisely because they flushed out differences of this kind.

Separate or shared management development?

The design of the workshops, with their subgroups of GPs only, practice managers only and mixed groups, offered opportunities for both separate and shared development. Mixed group learning offers GPs and practice managers the opportunity to see how GPs and practice managers outside their own practices function and how their own GP or practice manager colleague functions in a group outside the practice setting. When they come to an event together, they are subsequently able to debrief each other. This consolidates learning and enhances their understanding of each other's perspective. Mixed events also offer an arena in which issues can be raised that would be difficult to raise within the confines of the individual GP–practice manager relationship within the practice. They also enable GPs and practice managers to explore the shifting definitions between what is clinical and what is managerial, and how these two aspects of practice life intersect.

In some of the mixed groups, some practice managers were inhibited by the presence of GPs, although we always ensured that a GP–practice manager pair from the same practice were not in the same subgroup. In spite of this, some practice managers and some GPs objected to the separate subgroups, as they so valued the opportunity to hear and learn from each other's perspectives.

Practice managers in these workshops learned a great deal about what might be termed 'the current crisis in general practice (as a profession)' and the impact this has on practices as organizations. Similarly, GPs learned more about the emerging occupation of practice management and its impact on individual practice managers and the practices in which they work.

GPs and practice managers, however, appeared more able to voice their anxieties about their own GP–practice manager relationships and role conflicts when in separate groups. Some

GPs also used their separate GP groups to vent their anger, anxiety and despair about recent changes in the NHS, and to the GP contract in particular. They were feeling squeezed from the entry of nurse practitioners on one side and the outreach of specialist consultants on the other, in a context of increasing demands from the health commissions.

These discussions illustrated the need for GPs to be offered opportunities to develop a fuller understanding of health care trends nationally and internationally, and to work through their own personal and professional anxieties about these. Without such opportunities, they will remain defensive and resistant to delegation, whether clinical or managerial.

They also need opportunities to work through the medico-legal risks in delegation. This appeared as a central feature of their 'futures' and, when associated with increasing patient complaints, generates great anxiety. Until GPs have these opportunities, many will resist governmental or NHS managers' advocacy of primary care as the principal focus of responsibility for health and health care delivery.

They need structured opportunities to analyse and work through their feelings about:

- the GP role

- general practice as a profession

- general practice as an organization (the practice)

and how each influences the other, the environment and the individual GP. These opportunities are probably best offered through the postgraduate education system, but should include contributions from management and health policy academics, NHS and practice managers.

The 'separate or shared development' question can also be interpreted as a gender issue, and the specific needs of women practice managers have been emphasized throughout this book. The Women's Unit of the NHS Executive which co-sponsored the workshops on which this book is based is already supporting practice manager development. The problem for the Women's Unit and for other sponsors and providers of development programmes is that the title 'practice manager' currently covers a wide variety of people, functioning at very different levels of capacity and role. Consequently, provision of an adequate diagnostic service prior to provision of management development opportunity is crucial.

Practice managers pay a price for not being employees of the NHS, in the matter of superannuation which is now under discussion nationally, but also in relation to training and development. While FHSAs and health commissions have financed skills training, including assertiveness training, practice managers are not part of the networks used to publicize courses sponsored by the Women's Unit, nor are most of them readers of the *Health Service Journal* which advertises them.

The Women's Unit needs to work with the AMGP and IHSM to ensure that practice managers are aware of what is offered. Some practice managers wish to take part in wider NHS programmes and would bring to these high expectations. They would want to be stretched and to get a sense of how they shape up against managers outside general practice.

As managers of small businesses, they would also contribute a sharp sense of 'the bottom line' which has been slow to develop in NHS providers. Their presence would also alert NHS managers to the nature of independent contractor-based organizations which are becoming an increasing feature of the health and social care environment. There cannot be many women on the Opportunity 2000 programmes currently who are expected to manage the men who are also their employers.

Implications for management development providers

Because of the variety of management development needs, provision must be learner-centred and based upon an adequate diagnosis of individual need.

Whatever is provided must address learners' needs to understand and work through feelings about what many of them currently perceive to be enforced change, as well as their needs to manage it; indeed, the one is a precondition of the other. Many will continue to request training in management skills. Such requests are legitimate and must be met, but unless they are grounded in a deeper understanding of the changing local, national and international context to their work in health care, GPs and practice managers will continue to be unable and indeed unwilling to influence more broadly the direction of that health care.

Because of this, small group learning is the preferred mode. Existing groups established through AMGP or health commission networks for practice managers, and young principals' and trainers' groups for GPs could usefully be built upon. GPs and practice managers have limited time available, so that if existing support groups can also function well as learning groups through being better resourced, either through skilled facilitation or provision of learning materials, these should be provided.

Small groupwork is favoured because it offers opportunities to:

- share comparative experience

- share understanding, ideas and feelings

- co-consult on issues

- build interpractice networks.

Participants, particularly those in the middle ground of management awareness and expertise, wished to experience an integrated management development programme which would offer a diagnostic experience initially, followed by a modular programme that would allow for differences in areas and levels of expertise, linked perhaps by a learning set which would meet at regular intervals through the total time period taken to complete the programme.

Modules could be of two types:

1 seminars aimed at achieving a deeper understanding of both health policy nationally and internationally, and of new directions in management research and literature

2 workshops aimed at developing

- overall managerial competence

- enhanced GP–practice manager relationships

- specific skills demanded by the most recent legislation and policy directives.

In their learning sets, participants would be able to work through the personal issues arising from work in the modules. Such a programme could be designed for GPs alone, practice managers alone or GPs and practice managers together, and would typically be offered by a local university, college or the postgraduate education system, or collaboration between these and local funders such as the new health authorities.

Providers need to keep in mind the different needs of practice managers and GPs at different stages of their managerial development. Most GPs will never become managers. Before deciding what to provide for them, it is vital to clarify whether the GP wants *to learn about management, to learn to manage, to learn what and what not to manage, or to become a manager – or all of these.*

These distinctions affirm the importance of skilled diagnosis of GPs' management development needs and the need to ensure that development programmes are sufficiently flexible to take account of potential changes in aspiration and need over time. Over the past five years, much of the anger GPs feel towards government has been directed at NHS managers. Government policies throughout this period have aggravated GPs' negative stereotypes of organization and management that are inherent in their independent contractor identity. Once they experience the positive advantages of a well-managed practice and of the practice's capacity to influence the local direction of health care, these stereotypes begin to be questioned. Some GPs go further and find in management theory and practice an unexpected and pleasurable intellectual challenge.

Institutions which provide management development programmes specifically addressed to the development of practice-based primary care need also to understand the particular organizational nature of general practice and its implications for practice managers and for the GP–practice manager relationship. This understanding is enhanced if staff working on the programmes also work alongside GPs and practice managers as consultants.

Implications for funding

'It is how to still deliver personal, continuing care within the practice population framework. What's driving USA doctors is the same as here. How do I work in a managed service? What role do I take? Do I have a role?' (GP)

'Our management experience is very minimal; we did what the senior partner did and we learned a lot from the senior secretary who became the practice manager.' (GP, 45+)

'Ten to 15 years ago we were glorified secretaries. We feel GPs are recognizing practice manager status more now, we are being listened to more. Our ideas are being incorporated into practice plans now.' (practice manager)

'The health commission is helping us tremendously, organizing workshops like this and training programmes, so we don't want to see the end of that please.' (practice manager)

GPs and practice managers attending the workshops ranged in age from about 35 to 55 years, with the majority lying in the range 40–50 years. They will be working in primary care for a good many more years. If the NHS Executive and health commissions want to promote primary care development they have no alternative but to provide management development opportunities for these participants and others like them.

The GPs insisted that new money must be found for management development; it must not be funded from patient care allocations. Because increasing managerial demands were being made on GPs, both inside and outside the practice, these GPs felt they had less time available for clinical work. Locums would need to be provided if GPs were seriously to engage in management development activity. The postgraduate education allowance would not cover the costs. Attendance at the workshops was secured partly because locum payments were offered. Some GPs and practice managers also asked for the equivalent of locum cover for practice managers, as there was typically no one within the practice who could cover the practice manager's work.

A small minority of GPs were willing to pay a proportion of the costs of their own and their practice manager's development, in the belief that people value what they pay for and can demand more of providers if they pay.

The new health authorities could apply incentives to increase take-up of management development opportunities, through reimbursement of costs, regrading of practice managers who have undertaken management development and through resources for desired developments in the practice. They could also require, as a condition of funding the whole or part of a particular programme, such as an MBA or an Opportunity 2000 programme, submission of a report on the programme and agreement that the graduate be available for consultation by other managers or GPs who might wish to enter the programme.

Towards 2000 $\quad$ 8

General practice and the new health authorities

The workshops which provided much of the material for this book were conducted between October 1993 and March 1994 in two counties which were then part of Wessex Regional Health Authority. Although statutory DHAs and FHSAs remained, integrated health commissioning organizations had been formed across Wessex. In one county the FHSA and DHA were coterminous and came together in one building under one Chief Executive; in the other country, three health commissions were created in three DHA areas and incorporated various aspects of the FHSA's functions. The FHSA continued to exist in its own building quite separate from the three new Commissions. Not surprisingly, this arrangement proved far more difficult for GPs and practice managers to understand and they remained confused about the respective roles and responsibilities of the Commission and the FHSA.

Since these workshops were held, EL(94)79[40] has been issued, paving the way for the creation of new health authorities from April 1996 and accelerating the development of integrated organizational arrangements in those DHAs and FHSAs which have proceeded more slowly.

EL(94)79 states that a major role for the new authorities will lie in *developing primary care and forging a constructive partnership with GPs*. This role is elaborated under three headings:

- '*Strategy*. Health authorities will develop a strategy in collaboration with GPs, local people and other agencies (particularly local authorities) to meet national and local priorities . . .'

- '*Monitoring*. Within the national framework, health authorities will advise on budget allocations to GP fundholders and ensure that the way in which GPs fulfil their providing and purchasing role is in the interests of patients and local people. They will be responsible for ensuring that national policy and local strategy are implemented effectively.'

- '*Support*. Health authorities will provide support to GPs in both their primary care provision and fundholding capacities through the provision of advice, investment and training . . .'

The circular states that the role outlined above 'requires *all* health authorities to understand and support primary care provision, to work closely with fundholders and enable GPs to become fundholders, and to ensure all GPs contribute to the development of local strategy'.

Perceptions by GPs and practice managers of the emerging relationships between themselves and the Wessex Health Commissions at the time of the workshops offer some lessons which may be useful to those now engaged in creating the new health authorities.

Practices varied greatly from those which were still virtually one man (or woman) bands through to huge multi-partner, multi-site organizations with well over 20 000 patients.

Practice size is a major determinant of the pattern of practice organization and management, but within each size category there are significant exceptions to the general picture.

Overall, however, the majority of practices are small organizations of a type unfamiliar to most NHS managers on the DHA side. They are *both* small businesses *and* professional organizations, and each one strikes its own balance between the two. GPs participating in the workshops were attracted to a model of practice organization which defined the partnership as a board of directors and individual GPs as clinical members of the primary care team, accountable for the organizational aspects of their work to the practice manager. Not all were happy with this model, but it helped many GPs and practice managers to rethink their organization, their relationship, and their individual behaviour. Nevertheless, GPs are not only *doctors* and *directors*, but also *owners* of their organizations.

The more that GPs are helped to work through the distinctions between their managerial and their clinical roles, the easier it will be for health authorities to relate to and negotiate with them. At present, they slip from one to the other in the same conversation. In negotiations between health authorities and practices, health authority managers need to be clear whether they themselves are relating to the GPs as clinicians, as managers or as both.

When relating to 'the practice' as the providing and/or purchasing unit, it might also be helpful if health authority managers related to the GPs as directors and assumed that the practice manager would be present in any negotiations or discussions. This would signal to GPs the importance the health authority gives to effective practice management and managers.

NHS managers have largely responded well to the requirement to get closer to GPs. They have not been directed to get closer to practice managers, but in many practice managers they will find potential bridge builders between themselves and practices, and across different practices. Many practice managers have formed networks in which they are thinking through potential futures in primary care and considering how best they can help their organizations meet these. Health authorities should not underestimate the value of their perspective.

The new health authorities also need to do all they can to promote the development of effective practice management. This may not be achievable solely through the provision of education and development opportunities. Poor appointments continue to be made, often by those GPs in practices which would most benefit from the services of a capable practice manager who was enabled to practise as such. Health authorities need to think of ways in which they might influence this process in an encouraging and developmental rather than a controlling and regulatory manner. While health authority attempts to influence the appointment of practice-employed staff is a delicate issue, GPs will respond to incentives. Increasingly they themselves recognize that to survive and thrive in the new NHS they must achieve an effective and efficient organization.

In comparison to the stability of general practice over the previous 25 years, the years since 1989 have brought unremitting change not least in the terms of the GP contract, the development of fundholding and the development of new styles of management by FHSAs and health commissions. GPs and practice managers now face what they perceive to be the loss of 'their' health authorities, namely the FHSAs, and their replacement by new organizations with new management structures and cultures. Some GPs in the workshops felt hostile to the Wessex Health Commissions, particularly when they perceived their structures to be constantly changing. They would receive lists of managers' names and roles, but could attach little meaning to these without the opportunity for discussion.

Coming from small organizations which are very stable over time and which tend in some cases to resemble families rather than formal organizations, some GPs are naturally suspicious of large organizations. They trust individuals rather than organizations, and just as they value continuing personal relationships with patients and with hospital consultants, they also valued these with FHSA managers in the past.

If the NHS is to become primary-care-led, the new health authorities will need to build into their own organizations direct experience of management in practice-based primary care. One way of developing the capacity of both health authorities and practices is to encourage exchange or secondment of staff between the two. Although many GPs and practice managers would not be interested in such schemes, some certainly would and health authorities could gain significantly from them.

The organizational cultures of general practice and health commissions are very different. Both would benefit from the availability of a small cadre of people who know and have experience of both.

Research and development

The workshop discussions reported in this book repeatedly revealed the paucity of empirical research evidence on the rapid changes occurring in the organization of practice-based primary care. The pace of change is such that research appears to follow rather than inform its direction. This may be inevitable when the initiative for change has been deliberately passed to organizations led by independent contractors who have, although they may deny it, much freedom to develop those organizations as they wish.

Whereas many practices would still be recognizable to a time traveller from 50 let alone 20 years ago, some would not. These are evolving into primary care organizations that push the boundaries even of Pratt's 'practice' model of care[2]. While some of these organizational developments have been spurred by the introduction of fundholding, others have developed out of the entrepreneurialism and professionalism of GPs, and out of creative partnership between such GPs and health commissions[41]. They appear to be moving closer to the 'primary

managed care' model outlined by Nichol[24] and could be evaluated along some of its dimensions.

Like Pratt, Nichol poses the potential tension between
effectiveness and efficiency on the one hand and patient
preference on the other. It is always assumed, particularly by
GPs, that patients prefer personal continuity of care from a
particular doctor, however large and complex the practice
becomes. Certainly, some patients and some GPs seek to en-
shrine their preference in supporting the continuation of
single-handed practices, although even in these, if the GP is
supported by a primary care team, patients will on occasion be
treated and seen by its members. Meanwhile, in some of the
largest group practices, GPs retain the personal list system by
which patients enjoy personal continuing care from the same
doctor. Realistically, the more support the GP enjoys from
other clinically trained people within the team, the more
probable it is that on some visits to the practice the patient will
not see the GP at all.

Equally realistically, if GPs are to undertake the wider NHS
leadership role now being asked of them, their patients will
find that they are not always available within the practice. Does
this matter? Does it matter for some patients more than others,
for some patients *at certain times* or *in certain psychological states*?
Or can 'the organization' care? Can the new primary care
organizations manage themselves in such a way that 'the organization' itself is experienced as supportive and therapeutic?

Over the years, I have worked with practices that have been
perceived in this way by their patients. In 1970, an older patient
in London said to me, 'If a friend or neighbour comes to me
with a problem, I say "go to the Caversham, they'll help you"'.
A similar phrase was used in a suburb of Sydney in 1977 when
I evaluated the impact of a social worker's attachment to a
group practice[31]. Perhaps because of their more frequent
attendance for a range of needs, some older people build what
they perceive to be a personal relationship with 'the practice'
or 'medical centre'. They certainly become well-known to the
reception and nursing staff as well as to their doctor.

Both patients who made these comments to me enjoyed personal continuing care from the doctor of their choice within the practice, but also enjoyed what they experienced as *personalized* continuing care from *the organization*. It may be significant that both these organizations had a name by which they were known which did not relate to the names of any of the doctors practising in them. This sends an important signal to users of the organization and to other organizations which relate to it. It suggests that the practice as an organization is a reality and can be depended upon, and that a patient's attachment to it can be internalized by her as easily as she internalizes her relationship with her doctor.

We should not be surprised by this. We witness the same phenomenon when we see communities defend their local hospitals. The reason the London Teaching Hospitals are so difficult to close is that they have been internalized by both patients and staff. Identification is the most primitive kind of love and many people identify vigorously with their local hospitals, particularly if these have been the context for their own major life events such as birth, acute illness and death.

Traditionally, the primary care equivalent is perceived to be the doctor–patient relationship which has been the subject of much literature, fiction and non-fiction, autobiography and biography, as well as serious research. The practice as an organization has not stimulated the same kind of attention, perhaps because practices as organizations have traditionally been so small. Over the past 20 years, however, they have been growing rapidly, with a remarkable increase in those of over six partners[32]. National statistics of average practice size mask the development of practices such as the two represented in the Wessex workshops, which had well over 20 000 patients and over a dozen GPs working with a full complement of primary care nursing and other staff, with three or four premises each.

These practices could not have grown to this size unless they were attracting patients. How are they perceived by their patients? How do patients relate to these organizations? How do these organizations relate to their patients? What is it that some primary care organizations do that enables them to be experienced as helpful, caring and therapeutic in the way a person would be?

If the public, as well as GPs, is to accept the desirability of a primary-care-led NHS, these questions are in urgent need of an answer, for practice management is not just a business in which increasing numbers of people other than GPs have a stake. It is an activity which can either support and promote or subjugate or sabotage the therapeutic endeavour which lies at the heart of primary care.

Some practices are able to engage their populations in a shared therapeutic endeavour that embraces health promotion and disease prevention in the broadest sense as well as the care of those who are ill or believe themselves to be ill. These practices are held in deep regard by their communities. As yet we know even less about that relationship than we do about the relationship between individual patients and their practices.

If UK health care in the year 2000 is to be primary-care-led, perhaps those who manage R&D funding should make practice management very much their business.

Appendix I analysis of a survey of managers in general practice

This survey was based on the responses of 181 practice managers who were due to attend the Institute of Health Services Management/Radcliffe Practice Managers' Conference (July 1994), and was inserted in *Practice Manager*. Out of its circulation of over 6000, 503 practice managers completed all sections of the questionnaire. This cannot strictly be seen as a random sample of *all* practice managers, but the readership of *Practice Manager* does represent a good cross section.

Of these 503, 386 (77%) were female and 96 (19%) were male; a further 21 (4%) made no response to the gender question. Responses to some of the issues are analysed below.

Comparison by gender

While the highest priority overall was given to the issue of being *treated as professionals alongside others in the primary health care team*, this masked a major gender difference. For females this issue remained their highest priority, while males gave *terms, conditions, and salary commensurate to NHS* their highest rating.

Acceptability to clinicians (GPs and others) is a big issue for many practice managers, and is likely to be more keenly felt by those who identify strongly with the practice. To achieve status *inside* the practice, however, they may need to achieve it *outside*.

This realization is evident in their other priorities, especially those of the men. Male practice managers appear to be keener to identify themselves with the broader family of NHS managers; they want comparable conditions of work *and* greater involvement in NHS policy making. In this respect they constitute potential Trojan horses within the practice-based primary care sector whose culture has for so long been dominated by independent contractors who have jealously guarded their right to employ *their* staff.

The priority of making practice managers' and posts in the NHS interchangeable is one which only male respondents expressed, just as more of them wanted to see practice managers more involved in health service policy making. Male practice managers appear to see career horizons beyond the practice. They feel *entitled* to a place in the wider scheme of things, whereas some of the women still feel they lack a place in the sun, even within the narrower parameters of the practice itself. They feel more keenly the need to educate GPs as to their value, to introduce standards for practice managers and to have a clearly defined and recognized programme of training.

This may imply a female bias towards a stronger identification with the practice, simply because greater numbers of them have come through the practice staff ranks. In 1994 the Association of Health Centre and Practice Administrators (AHCPA), renamed itself the Association of Managers in General Practice, thereby affirming its primary identification. The Association has until very recently been not just an association of practice managers but an association of women, which led and supported the aspirations of many practice managers who were determined to grow with and through the changes in the job.

The Association's key themes in recent years have been the definition of the practice manager role, recognized qualifications for practice managers and the establishment of clearly defined and recognized programmes of training. These are all reflected in the issues rated more highly by women in the IHSM survey.

Comparison by annual salary

The data showed that the *need to educate GPs as to our value* was not a priority at all for practice managers paid over £30 000. They had presumably already achieved this objective. They also set small store on being *treated as professionals alongside others in the primary care team*, feeling that their salary reflected their status. They make their highest priorities *a national strategy for resourcing practice manager development* and *practice managers more involved in NHS policy making*. There are leaders here, and leaders who are not content to confine their influence within their practices.

The NHS is currently missing out on the ideas and insights of these potential Trojan horses who have entered the terrain that remains so foreign to most NHS managers. The workshop experiences reported in this book suggest that many practice managers who enter practice from business, commerce, the armed forces, and indeed other parts of the NHS, question what they see in practice-based primary care. Some GPs are brave enough to recruit them for just this capacity: being far-sighted, they value a critical appraisal of their business and consequent proposals for change. They sense this may enable them not only to survive but to thrive in the new NHS.

The survey's commentary suggests that the less the annual salary respondents earn, the more they want 'GPs to be educated as to their value'. One could question why, if they have not convinced their GPs of their value, they should be paid more; alternatively, should they seek employment which would reward them more handsomely? Many practice managers are remarkably resistant to moving. This 'culture of loyalty' extracts a high price from practice managers. It also does the service no favours, for it frequently masks managerial stalemate in the practice.

Major areas of responsibility

The data show that for almost 91% of respondents *personnel and training* was the major area of responsibility, with *general administration, practice finance, health and safety, and premises* running very close. By contrast, *business planning, surgery, and audit* were stated as major areas by only 60% of respondents.

A much smaller percentage stated that *contract negotiation, fund management, and health care purchasing and strategies* were major areas of responsibility, perhaps not surprisingly as these are more associated with fundholding practices and these currently represent only 30% of all practices.

A good 30% of practice managers appear not to be involved in any major way with the strategic development of the practice and with quality. This is not surprising, but is a cause for concern. It is very difficult for practice managers who have been appointed from receptionist or secretarial positions within the practice to *push* GPs into these areas or to enter the areas themselves without GP support. Many of these internal recruits to practice management are oversocialized into the existing culture of the practice, including its hierarchical aspects. New entrants, particularly men and particularly people (of either gender) who enter from *established managerial careers outside*, do not usually don the mantle of deference as they enter the practice, but view both GPs and themselves as complementary professionals.

Careers

The data indicating the *job held before becoming a practice manager* might surprise those who assume that most practice managers have been promoted from within. Whereas 38% were previously receptionists or practice administrators, 54% were managers in the NHS, in non-health industry or 'other', which presumably would include those entering from the armed services. These 'others' and those from non-health industry comprise 45.8% of the total sample, which suggests that a large number of practices now contain potential agents for change. Some of these will be early retirees or those made redundant in other sectors of the economy who get a new lease of life from a new career. Others may be so damaged or burnt out that they have little to offer but a safe administrative pair of hands.

These data are not cross-tabulated with responses to the question 'How long have you been working in practice management?' but we can assume that there would be a high level of correspondence between them. Practice managers who were appointed from within the practice will usually have worked in practice management for longer than those who have come in from other fields.

The real cause for concern in these data lies in the tiny proportion (8.3%) of the total who have come in from other parts of the Health Service. The inability to transfer conditions of work from the NHS into practice-based employment currently inhibits cross-fertilization of experience and expertise, and the development of a common culture.

Training

The data analyse the feelings of practice managers about adequacy of training for the role, access to training and sense of FHSA support for practice manager training and development. Over 73% of managers felt adequately trained to carry out their current role which was matched by 78% who felt their local FHSA/commission/board was supportive of practice manager training and development. Over 16% of managers did not, however, feel adequately trained for their *current* role, and 17% did not feel they had access to training for their *changing* role in the future of primary care.

Whereas almost 80% of FHSAs/commissions/boards are perceived to support practice manager training and development, 11% of managers feel that their local FHSA/commission/board is not supportive. A further 8% neither agreed nor disagreed on this statement. Over 74% reported that they had access to training funds from the FHSA/commission/board, whereas almost 20% reported that they did not.

Whereas 56% of managers reported that their practices had a training budget for staff, over 46% were unable to identify the amount. About 20% said less than £1000, 23% between £1000 and £2500, 8% between £2501 and £5000 and 1.6% over £5000. These are training budgets for *all* staff excluding GPs, and only 10% were over £2501.

If the NHS is to achieve the strategic shift to primary care, practices will need to develop the organizational and managerial capacity not only to cope but to lead. Practice managers are pivotal in achieving this change in practice capacity, but will need considerable support. Management education and development is a costly commodity, particularly when so much of what is available derives from organizational models which are radically different from that of general practice.

Practice managers, like GPs, are thus faced with a 'translation' process that is not easy and for which they need considerable support. This book has insisted that skills training is not sufficient and that practice managers need a deeper understanding of health policy and of modern management as a context for skill development, while those who are also women require programmes which offer personal as well as professional development.

Without this investment the strategic shift will remain rhetoric rather than reality.

Appendix II participants' proposals for management development activities

Global management skills for GPs

What we need

- improve understanding
- really know our feelings
- delegate appropriately
- development thereafter
- expand horizons (work outside, e.g. health commission)
- develop within ourselves and within practice
- financial gain for completion and implementation of course, e.g. re-accreditation money.

Why

- have to!
- self-employed therefore self-imposed (to an extent)

- dichotomy: caring professional versus business person
- crossroads – we choose/need to maintain autonomy (alternative salaried GPs)
- build flexibility (too cumbersome system).

Aims

- to generate FUN and FUNDS
- to improve our management potential (skills, capability, capacity)
- to discover the next stage of evolution within ourselves and therefore our practices for the benefit of ourselves, our patients and our practice (and thence the health authorities).

Content

- demystification of jargon and of content
- how to relate improved management skills to practice
- listening skills
- negotiating skills (understand NHS structure): Intrapartnership negotiation; interpartnership negotiation
- personal time management
- interviewing technique
- hiring, firing, appraisals, employment law, motivating
- delegating (practice manager and staff/GPs)
- finance, taxation; personal, practice, fundholding
- group dynamics (plus basic psychology)

- our own feelings in management and how we deal with personal conflicts, etc.

- relaxation skills.

NB: there is considerable overlap with practice managers, our brief was for GPs only.

Method

- FUN

- short lectures (20 min maximum)

- video/reading lists (John Cleese)

- small groups

- role play and feedback

- beware phobias: business management; partners' fears

- homework (not too much – some already available)

- end point (± certification)

- avoid 'diplomatosis'

- modules

- on site training

  - other practices

  - health commission

  - ICI boardroom

  - within practice

  - management consultant/trainer who keeps an eye on the practice

- running series of workshops (ongoing) and modular (so you can click in and out).

Timing

- must be protected time, i.e. working time, otherwise GPs would not attend (particularly the women); must not be seen as extra to GPs' load (NB: not truly self employed, not truly salaried – a hybrid, so protected time please)

- ballpark length of course:

  - one day per month and one residential course

  - modules that are repeated

  - as a foundation course which could go on to 'masters' equivalent (i.e. tiers – basic, basic plus, masters)

  - to prevent a new breed of 'senior partners' all partners should have the basic grounding course.

Funding/sponsorship

- new money (such as fundholding management allowance which is directly Treasury)

- not from NHS budget

- not from patient care

- not from RCGP

- possible sponsors: RCGP, Wessex Trust, health commission, Regional Health Authority to 1996; drug companies, BUPA.

A structured approach to the development of practice managers/practice management

Aim

- structured career development of managers linked with practice development.

Objectives

- to improve confidence in manager and others in the practice team
- to make explicit the direction of the practice, thereby identifying training needs, e.g. communication.

Who for?

- whoever is managing the practice, practice manager/GP.

Method

- diagnostic for
  - manager
  - practice team
  - needs of geographical area (localized)
- positive feedback; then personal and practice plans for training

- diagnostic event annually ('away day'), initial diagnostic event may need to be longer, to be delivered within local area (less than 1 hour drive)
- training: half to full day sessions, one subject at a time plus time to reflect/think; review and follow-up; evaluation plan – personal/practice
- must be interactive, e.g. effective listening.

Frequency

- short course over 6–8 weeks, longer subjects quarterly, run side by side.

Personal development diagnosis

- regular reviews
- a body to help with this process, not necessarily FHSA/ health commissions.

Practice development diagnosis

- review other members of team
- needs time and resources
- practice supporting practice manager following course – time implications
- structured system of obtaining practice manager's views of their needs
- course component to be structured to enable practice managers to dip into/out of
- practical evaluation of benefit

- forum available to practice managers to share information
- should connect with current demands, e.g. half-yearly health promotion report.

Sponsorship

- funding – jointly health commissions and practice
- running it
    - independent body for diagnostic local training needs
    - other bodies providing specifics (could be practice managers/FHSA/health commissions, local trusts; need fuller information on local providers' offerings)
- mentorship very important; not within the practice because of size (1–3 partners is too small) but would like interest shown
- mentor could come from another practice, FHSA/health commission/trust.

An educational event/programme for locality group members

(The account presented here does not do justice to the reporting GPs' 'mapped' record of the discussion.)

Aims of the educational process

- to get our act together
- to develop a structure
- empowerment

- to involve as many as possible of those eligible
- to be responsive to members' needs
- what would/should locality group provide?
- to establish the role for the group
- to make effective and continuing group
- ?separate meeting for leaders
- to encourage openness – acknowledge fears/threats
- to look at group's development/future and to enable this.

Content

- locality health plans
- group leadership, chairmanship, meeting skills
- decide whether to consider priorities
- funding of group
- fairness of representation
- linking back to practice
- decision making/negotiation, e.g. what services? where?
- consensus, loss of autonomy/ownership, competition, confidentiality – feelings associated with these
- information sharing
- context and environment.

Who

- locality group members
  - GPs: all, some, key people, leaders

- practice managers
- secretary; to record decisions
- teachers: health service, education, business
- others' views, e.g. health commission.

How

- as part of existing meeting, this/these meetings can model good practice: well run groups, well managed meetings, rules, e.g. confronting, respect, etc.
- and/or as a separate meeting/ongoing process
- learning by doing: facilitator essential.

Where

- comfortable
- suitable facilities
- convenient
- neutral ground or rotating
- cost.

When

- convenient time for majority
- protected time at least for initial meeting
- working day.

Funding/sponsorship

- FHSA/health commission
- regional primary care R&D
- Postgraduate Education Authority (PGEA) accreditation
- to remove disincentives to attend
- central government
- anyone who believes locality groups will improve patient care!

Locality groups

- Function
  - cheaper option
  - alternative to two tiers
  - feedback to purchasers
  - response to fundholding
  - 'clout'
  - representation of smaller practices
  - a pressure group, a consortium
  - ?tool to manage change – for DHC
  - ?to influence purchase of secondary care
  - to purchase services
  - to provide services
- Issues
  - confidentiality/competition/local cooperation, etc. arising, e.g. in linking practice health plans to locality health plans

- representation/equity in view of variety of practice size
- communication and crossover: Local Medical Committee, Community Medical Committee, health commission; non-fundholding group,CMC, core groups
- hidden agenda: bypass existing structures?
- structure: manager, secretarial support, decision making.

'Are you getting the best out of your practice manager?'

A proposal for a half-day workshop for GPs.

Why?

- doctors have all the responsibility and not necessarily the skills
- practice managers have skills and responsibilities but little authority.

Method

- to be run by an experienced practice manager and GP pair (modelling a good working relationship)
- use case studies for discussion based on real experiences from practices, e.g. partners make a decision that would affect staff and ask practice manager to implement it; staff go behind practice manager's back to object, and GPs take the issue on board; representation of the practice with external bodies (health commission, accountant, trusts, etc.) could be prepared cases or examples brought by participants
- cases could be role-played.

References

1 Marsh GN (1991) *Efficient care in general practice.* Oxford University Press, London.

2 Pratt J (1995) *Practitioners and practices: a conflict of values?* Radcliffe Medical Press, Oxford.

3 Huntington J (1992) Some very peculiar practices. *Health Service Journal.* **105**: 5295:19.

4 Teasdale S (1992) Management and administration. *BMJ* **305**: 454–6.

5 Foster R (1994) Practice manager: a developing role. *Practice Nursing.* **515**: 18–20.

6 Jones RVH *et al.* (1978) *Running a practice.* Croom Helm, London.

7 Pritchard PMM *et al.* (1984) *Management in general practice.* Oxford University Press, London.

8 Hasler J *et al.* (1991) *Handbook of practice management.* Churchill Livingstone, London.

9   Houghton K (1991) *Practice Manager Development, Part One.* Radcliffe Medical Press, Oxford.

10 Griffiths R (1983) *NHS Management Inquiry Report.* DHSS, London.

11 Pollitt C (1990) *Managerialism and the public services: the Anglo-American Experience.* Blackwell, Oxford.

12 Harrison S *et al.* (1992) *Just managing: power and culture in the NHS.* Macmillan, London.

13 Department of Health and Social Security (1989) *Working for patients.* HMSO, London.

14 Royal College of General Practitioners (1987) *The front line of the health service: college response to primary care – an agenda for discussion, Report from General Practice No. 25.* RCGP, London.

15 Hasenfeld Y (1992) *Human services as complex organizations.* Sage, London.

16 Mattinson J and Sinclair I (1981) *Mate and stalemate: working with marital problems in a social services department.* Blackwell, Oxford.

17 Menzies Lyth I (1988) *Containing anxiety in institutions,* Vol. 1. Free Association Books, London.

18 Obholzer A and Roberts VZ (eds) (1994) *The unconscious at work.* Routledge, London.

19 Argyris C (1985) *Strategy change and defensive routines.* Pitman, London.

20 Balint M (1964) *The doctor, his patient, and the illness.* Pitman Medical, London.

21 Broadbent J (1994) *Practice managers and practice nurses: gatekeepers and handmaidens? A consideration of the effects of the new*

general practitioner contract (draft, personal communication from the author).

22 Huntington J *et al.* (1989) *We need a practice manager.* Video and coursebook pack produced for the RCGP by the MSD Foundation. Royal College of General Practitioners, London.

23 Royal College of General Practitioners and MSD Foundation (1992) *Partnership: can we talk?* Video and coursebook pack. Royal College of General Practitioners, London.

24 Nichol D (1994) Next steps for purchasing? Population and personalised care management. In Health Services Management Unit *Best practice in health care commissioning,* release 4, pp. 2.11.1–2.11.8. Churchill Livingstone, London.

25 Brownhill L and Marshall P (1993) Firm but unfair? *Health Service Journal.* **104:** 5394: 28–29.

26 Lawrence WG (ed.) (1979) *Exploring individual and organisational boundaries: a Tavistock open systems approach.* John Wiley & Sons, London.

27 Kahn RL *et al.* (1977) *Organisational stress: studies in role conflict and ambiguity.* John Wiley & Sons, London.

28 Senge P (1992) *The fifth discipline: the art and practice of the learning organisation.* Century Business, London.

29 Marsh GN and Kaim-Caudle P (1976) *Team care in general practice.* Croom Helm, London.

30 Bowling A and Stilwell B (1988) *The nurse in family practice.* Scutari, London.

31 Huntington J (1981) *Social work and general medical practice: collaboration or conflict?* George Allen & Unwin, London.

32 Fry J (1993) *General practice: the facts.* Radcliffe Medical Press, London.

33 NHS Executive (1995) *Education and Training in the new NHS,* EL(95)27. NHS Executive Headquarters, Leeds.

34 Advertisement (1994) *Health Service Journal.* **104:** 5398: 56.

35 Meads G (ed.) (Forthcoming) *Future options for general practice.* Radcliffe Medical Press, Oxford.

36 *Shorter English Oxford Dictionary,* Vol. 1. (1973) Oxford University Press, London.

37 National Association of Health Authorities and Trusts (NAHAT) (1994) *Partners in learning: developing postgraduate education for general practice.* NAHAT, Birmingham.

38 Royal College of General Practitioners (RCGP) (1994) *Education and training for general practice* (Proposed College Policy Statement – draft). RCGP, London.

39 Millar B (1994) Everything's coming up rosie. *Health Service Journal.* **104:** 5398: 12–13.

40 NHS Executive (1994) *Developing NHS purchasing and GP fundholding, EL(94)79.* NHS Executive Headquarters, Leeds.

41 Robinson B (1993) Lyme cordial. *Health Service Journal.* **103:** 5364: 20.

Index